Advance Praise for *Love Worth Making*

"*Love Worth Making* is, hands down the most practical, fun, and empowering book I've ever read on how to have a fabulous sex life in a committed relationship. It should be must reading for every committed couple who wants to keep the spark alive for many years." —Christiane Northrup, M.D., *New York Times* bestselling author of *Goddesses Never Age* and *The Wisdom of Menopause*

"A must-read for therapists who are not sex experts, this book is a guided tour of what happens when sex falls apart, and how to put it back together again." —Susan C. Vaughan, M.D., director of the Columbia University Center for Psychoanalytic Training and Research and author of *The Talking Cure*

"Mandatory reading for anyone who wants a better understanding of what the other sex is thinking in the bedroom." —Debra W. Soh, Ph.D., sex columnist at Playboy.com

"Master sex therapist Dr. Stephen Snyder takes us beneath the surface to the complex emotions and vulnerabilities that inhabit our sexual underground, then brings us back up again to connect with our true sexual selves." —Ian Kerner, Ph.D. LMFT, and *New York Times* bestselling author of *She Comes First*

"Most sex advice in books and on the internet today is wrong. Dr. Snyder explains why. There are at least ten core concepts here that will motivate and empower couples everywhere—including some that are unique and not found anywhere else." —Barry McCarthy, Ph.D., professor of psychology at American University and author of *Rekindling Desire*

"Dr. Snyder reminds us that in marriage, it is not new toys or novel positions but feelings that are the final erotic frontier."
—Peggy J. Kleinplatz, Ph.D., professor and director of sex and couples therapy training at the University of Ottawa, Canada

"I have very rarely been so impressed with the practicality and engagement of a couples' guide to maintaining long-term intimacy. Dr. Snyder's approach is incredibly compelling and will serve readers of this book well. I am so glad he has made his work available to all." —Kat Van Kirk, Ph.D., author of *The Married Sex Solution: A Realistic Guide to Saving Your Sex Life*

"What Dr. Snyder shows us is that the best sex is in a committed relationship, and that working together, couples can have the best sex imaginable—and he gives multiple suggestions on how to achieve that. I would highly recommend his book to my patients who really want the joys of a long-term relationship, and want to have continued fabulous sex." —Mary Jane Minkin, M.D., clinical professor in the Department of Obstetrics, Gynecology, and Reproductive Sciences at Yale Medical School

"Covers everything from how to know if you're really excited (it's not what you think) to how to handle the sexual consequences of your husband's ADHD. This book is one I'll be recommending to colleagues and clients for many years to come." —Lori Gottlieb, psychotherapist, *New York Times* bestselling author of *Marry Him* and *New York* magazine's "What Your Therapist Really Thinks" Columnist

LOVE
WORTH
MAKING

LOVE WORTH MAKING

HOW TO HAVE RIDICULOUSLY GREAT SEX IN A LONG-LASTING RELATIONSHIP

Stephen Snyder, M.D.

St. Martin's Press ⋈ New York

Note:

All stories in this book are composite, fictional accounts based on the experiences of many individuals. Similarities to any real person or persons are coincidental and unintentional.

This book is not intended as a manual for how to do sex therapy, nor is it intended to replace the advice of the reader's own physician or other licensed health professional. Individual readers are solely responsible for their own health care decisions and should consult a licensed health professional in such matters. The author and publisher do not accept responsibility for any adverse effects individuals may claim to experience, whether directly or indirectly, from the information contained in this book.

LOVE WORTH MAKING. Copyright © 2018 by Stephen Snyder. All rights reserved. Printed in the United States of America. For information, address St. Martin's Press, 175 Fifth Avenue, New York, N.Y. 10010.

www.stmartins.com

The Library of Congress Cataloging-in-Publication Data is available upon request.

ISBN 978-1-250-11311-5 (hardcover)
ISBN 978-1-250-11312-2 (ebook)

Our books may be purchased in bulk for promotional, educational, or business use. Please contact your local bookseller or the Macmillan Corporate and Premium Sales Department at 1-800-221-7945, extension 5442, or by email at MacmillanSpecialMarkets@macmillan.com.

First Edition: February 2018

10 9 8 7 6 5 4 3 2 1

We are like islands in the sea, separate on the surface but connected in the deep.

—WILLIAM JAMES

Contents

INTRODUCTION

Your Wife Is Not
a Lawn Mower

"Tell me about foreplay," I say to the next couple in my office. "What kind of foreplay do the two of you enjoy the most?"

"Well, we kiss," she says. "Then I touch him, and he touches me."

She's obviously speaking in some kind of secret code here. But you get the picture, right? She strokes his penis, and then he does something to her vulva with his hands.

Is this a good idea? Well, that depends. If this couple is riding a wave of ecstasy fueled by erotic touch, then sure. But in that case, chances are they wouldn't be sitting in my office.

More likely, they're just trying to get the job done—to get him hard and her wet, so they can have sex.

How many couples do it this way when they first fall in love? Not many. When passion is high, no one needs friction to get excited. Hardness and wetness just happen as effortlessly as the blooming of a flower.

That's the way it's supposed to go. The sexual self saying yes, in the only language it knows. Trying to convert a "no" to a "yes" by friction alone is like trying to convince a child he likes broccoli.

Forget it. It's not going to work. Friction may get you sex, but never good sex.

As I sit with this couple, I can't help recalling a scene from my suburban childhood—watching one of the neighborhood dads try to start up his gas lawn mower. You had to pull the cord just right for the engine to start, and this took practice and skill.

I live in Manhattan now where we don't have lawns. But the image is still stuck in my head—the mower, the cord, and the look of frustration on the face of the guy hoping to start the thing up.

I wonder whether this couple is old enough to have ever seen a gas mower.

"Look," I say to him. "Your wife is not a lawn mower. It's not just a question of pulling the cord right."

They both laugh.

"But how do I get her wet?" he asks.

"Simple. You don't."

He looks at me with curiosity.

"It's not your job to get her wet," I say. "Just enjoy your own excitement, and let her enjoy hers."

"That doesn't sound very romantic."

"It's actually *much more romantic*, if you do it right. And something even more important."

"What's that?" he asks.

"It's more *erotic*."

~~

These are astonishing times for sex. You can find new sex partners on your smartphone in minutes. Pornography is everywhere. And even kids in middle school know that if an erection lasts more than four hours you should call your doctor.

With a click of the mouse you can find new sex positions online, buy the latest vibrator, and learn the names for sex acts your grandparents never knew existed.

But with sex getting all this attention these days, are people feeling any more satisfied in bed?

I doubt it.

They know more sex techniques. And they certainly have more access to sex toys and other forms of erotic novelty. But if my experience is any guide, that's not what most people are really interested in.

What *are* they really interested in?

Simple:

They're interested in *relationships*. They want to have great sex in a committed relationship. They want sex to be an instrument of sanctification and peace at the center of a loving partnership.

You could look for a long time online and not find any deep secrets for how to do that.

It's no mystery why: The secrets to great sex in a committed relationship are largely emotional. And emotions are slippery things—hard to capture and sometimes even harder to communicate.

You could learn all about the best sex techniques, the latest scientific studies, and the newest kinky ways to stretch your erotic boundaries. But if all you really want to know is how to have great sex with someone you care about, then all the technical expertise, sexual science, and erotic novelty in the world probably aren't going to help you very much.

For that, you need something else:

You need to understand sexual feelings. How they operate, what rules they follow, and how they connect to the rest of who you are.

~

This is a book about sexual feelings.

It's unabashedly about sex—as you'll see. But it has much to do with erotic love as well. Its main concerns are more emotional than physical.

This is not a book about how to turn your partner on. It's not about how to give someone the world's greatest orgasm. Instead, it's about coming home to yourself as a sexual person.

You might say it's about finding your sexual heart. Once you've found your sexual heart, those other details tend not to matter so much.

Over the last thirty years, I've treated over fifteen hundred individuals and couples using the methods you're going to read about here. I know this approach helps people. And I'm confident that no matter where you're starting from, it can help you connect more deeply with your sexual feelings and enjoy them for life.

PART I

Your Sexual Self

This is a book about good sex, bad sex, and great sex—from someone who's heard his share about all kinds.

In Part I, we'll consider some of the basic rules for good sex. You might be surprised to find these have nothing to do with hardness, wetness, intercourse, or orgasm—although those things often go much better if you're paying attention to the rules I'm going to tell you about.

Along the way, I'll describe the core attributes of what many people in the sex field call the "sexual self." This is an intuitive concept, and is purely subjective. It's not based on any known science. You'll either feel the truth of what I'm saying, or you won't.

The rules that I have in mind are exceptionally easy to follow, once you understand them. They all involve staying out of your own way, so your sexual self can do what it knows how to do naturally.

Some of what you'll read here will seem familiar. And some will almost certainly surprise you. But I'm pretty sure you'll come away with a clearer idea of what really matters in lovemaking—and how you and the person next to you in bed can get more of the stuff that counts.

1

Rules of the Heart

The rules of desire are rules of the heart.

"Sex is emotion in motion."
—MAE WEST

It's a hot summer afternoon on the New York subway. I'm bringing my children and a few of their friends back to Manhattan on the B train after a long day at Brighton Beach.

There's a young couple standing near the exit door sharing an iPod headset—tethered together, each with an earpiece in one ear. She's leaning against the wall, sweat-soaked in a T-shirt and shorts. He's a few inches shorter, wearing sandals, beach clothes, and long hair. His hands are resting lightly on her hips. Her arms are draped over his shoulders.

They seem entirely absorbed in the music, the motion of the subway car, and each other. Their eyes, half shut, are out of focus, dreamy. They're both wearing goofy, crooked smiles—as if sharing some silly secret. They look as if they might easily miss their stop.

Amid the noise of the children and the rocking and bouncing of the subway car, it would be easy for this couple to pass unnoticed. But there is something about them that holds my attention. A certain aura.

~~

It's sex, of course.

Their goofy smiles, their dreamy manner. Definitely sex.

They're fully clothed, standing up, and doing nothing obviously improper, but definitely enjoying a long moment of arousal on the way home from the beach.

Turning away self-consciously, I realize I'm not the only one watching this couple. The young children are oblivious, of course. But the adults in the car are all clearly aware of what's going on. Everyone is stealing glances at them, transfixed by the same sexual vibration.

Their aura is now general throughout the subway car. I fear we will all miss our stops.

~~

Sexual arousal, if all goes according to nature's plan, makes us dumb and happy, absorbed and distracted. We arrive somewhere far uptown, having missed all our stops—deeply pleasured but with no idea where we are.

Most of us learn that to succeed in a fast-paced world we don't really have time for arousal. Many modern couples hurry through sex without letting themselves get very aroused—then wonder where their sexual magic has gone. Others do their best to hold on to the inspiration that brought them together, but lose it amid the distractions and responsibilities of ordinary adult life.

Eros seems more designed to get you *into* a relationship than to keep you happy once you're already there. This young couple quietly rocking near the exit door—if they stay together, what will their lovemaking be like years from now, when they're the ones lugging kids' swim toys back from the beach?

Looking around the subway car, I find myself wondering about the sex lives of my fellow passengers. Who's having good sex, and who isn't? Who's faking it, and whose bedroom is still a sanctuary of delight?

Our intimate lives are conducted almost entirely in secret. No one except you and your partner really know what your erotic life is like—unless one of you tells, of course. And even then, things often get lost in translation.

Some people know intuitively how to cultivate a vibrant erotic relationship. But many don't. Which is unfortunate, since it's actually not that hard—once you know what you're doing.

A Funny Story

One day in sixth grade, my daughter came home from school with a funny story. Her teacher had been going around the room asking each student what her parents did for a living.

When it came my daughter's turn to tell about me, she said I was a psychiatrist. Whereupon her best friend seated behind her shouted, *"He's a sex therapist!"*

The class went wild.

A few minutes later, when all the shouting and excitement had died down, one classmate whispered aloud the inevitable question . . .

"What does he . . . DO?"

There was much wonderment, horror, and giggling.

It's a good question, really. Since 1978, when the American Association of Sex Educators, Counselors, and Therapists (AASECT) prohibited nudity and physical touch in the office, it's assumed that all we do is talk. For the most part that's true.

We talk about sex, of course. But we talk even more about feelings. Spend enough time as a sex therapist, and before long you're either doing psychotherapy or you haven't been paying attention.

Sometimes when I'm asked "What does a sex therapist do?" I'm tempted to give a much simpler answer. One that I'm sure would have been both a relief and a disappointment to my daughters' class-mates:

Mostly I listen to people tell me about bad sex.

In my thirty years of practice, I've heard about more bad sex than you can possibly imagine. In fact, by now I feel I can without exaggeration claim to be one of the world's foremost experts on bad sex.

I know that sounds like a dubious honor. But being an expert on bad sex can be really useful. Listening to people tell me about bad sex for so many years has left me with a deeper understanding about what makes for *good sex*—and even *great* sex.

The Rules of Desire

Good sex follows certain rules. The same is true for great sex.

Some people know these rules intuitively, but many don't. I know this for a fact because every day in my office I see couples who have no idea such rules even exist.

Most therapists don't know these rules either. For example, I'll sometimes hear a colleague remark that sex is simply "friction plus fantasy." Sexual excitement, they say, happens when you combine the right kind of physical stimulation with the right kind of mental activity.

This tells me right away that my colleague is unaware of the rules.

I have nothing against friction and fantasy. But if that's all you're getting, then you've been short-changed.

Good friction is nice—and certainly better than bad friction. But friction doesn't really do the trick—as anyone who's ever had really boring sex with a really skilled partner can tell you.

Think back to the most memorable sexual experience of your life. (If you've never yet *had* a really memorable sexual experience, relax. You're in good company.) What you remember probably isn't how wonderful the friction was.

The rules I have in mind don't involve sexual friction.

How about the *fantasy* part of the "friction plus fantasy" equation? There's very little that happens to us humans without our automatically adding to it from our store of memories, dreams, and associations. So of course we fantasize during sex as well.

We may or may not go so far as to imagine alternate partners in bed, but one would have to search hard for examples of sex where fantasy was entirely absent.

The power of fantasy tends to be fleeting though. The mind is a restless consumer, always looking for something new and wondering, "Is that all there is?"

The rules I have in mind don't involve sexual fantasy either.

A Hidden Realm

Somewhere beyond "friction plus fantasy" is a realm where sexuality connects us to each other and to the deepest parts of ourselves. It's a place where sex feeds and is fed by love.

This is the most personal aspect of sex. In all the many books that have been written on lovemaking, you'll find precious little written about it.

It's no mystery why. This aspect of sex is not an easy subject. But this "sex of the heart" is an essential subject if you want to understand lovemaking.

It's in this realm of sex of the heart that we'll find the hidden rules we're seeking.

Most of us feel this more personal erotic feeling somewhere in our chests. Hence, by tradition, "heart." A more precise term, though lacking in physical resonance, might be "sex of the self."

Unlike friction and fantasy, this part of sex can't be bought, sold, marketed, or packaged as a commodity. It is simply a gift to be received. Its proper accompanying emotion is not really desire, or lust—but rather simply gratitude, or perhaps awe.

This kind of sex can't be produced simply by following a recipe. So it's no accident that few how-to books on sex concern themselves much with it.

Sex becomes truly special either of its own volition, or not at all. But we can help nurture the conditions for it to flourish, once we know what those conditions are.

Some Open Secrets About Sexual Arousal

In the late 1950s, William Masters and Virginia Johnson became the first scientists to examine the physical aspects of human sexual response in any detail. But many of these physical signs had already been closely observed—less scientifically but no less intensely—by millions of sexual couples since the dawn of human self-awareness.

Most couples study the male partner's erections and the female partner's state of lubrication carefully, for information about whether the other person is "really aroused." Urban legends rise and fall concerning other supposed indicators (see "nipple erection," "pupil dilation"). But this is all still limited to physical arousal.

The *psychological* aspects of arousal are more important. But they've yet to find their Masters and Johnson.

Fortunately, your own feelings can be a quite accurate guide to how excited you are—if you know what to look for.

Here's my short list of the most important psychological changes that happen when you get aroused.

Attention

When you're aroused, sex grabs your attention. You stop thinking about bills, worries, responsibilities—your entire portfolio of ordinary concerns. Your time sense may get a little messed up. (Sexually aroused people tend to arrive late to meetings.)

If someone gave you an IQ test during peak arousal, you wouldn't do too well on it. The tester might have a hard time getting you to pay attention to the questions. Good sex definitely makes you dumber. And great sex can make you downright stupid.

Regression

Sexual excitement puts you into a more primitive and selfish state of mind. It makes you less patient, less forgiving. You don't tolerate frustration very well. You become somewhat immature. (Okay, sometimes *a lot* immature!)

If the phone rings during lovemaking, you don't care who's calling, or what they want. You may feel very close to your partner, but it's a selfish kind of closeness. You're not really interested in listening to the details of how their day went. You just want them to give you their complete attention, and to tell you how wonderful you are.

Validation

Arousal feels special. Validating. Good sex makes us feel good about ourselves. That's how we know it's good sex.

With good lovemaking, we have a feeling of "Yes, that's me. Here I am. You found me." We feel in touch with our deepest, most authentic selves.

It's a grateful feeling. "Yes, you found me. The *me* of me. Thank you for finding me. Thank you for bringing me home to where I really live."

When couples come to my office, I always try to find out whether they've been really getting aroused. Not just hard, or lubricated. But really *aroused*. Captivated. Absorbed. *Self-absorbed*. Goofy. I like to hear a few giggles.

How to Use This Book

You'll find the rules I've been referring to at the beginning of every chapter, in italics. At the top of Chapter 2, for instance: *The sexual self is very honest, but its vocabulary is limited.*

Occasionally you'll find them other places in the text as well.

If you skim a few of them, you'll notice they're less like rules of conduct and more like the law of gravity. They're not so much to be followed as to be understood.

Feel free to go ahead and break them. But if you do, please write me and tell me how you did it.

This is not a conventional "how-to" book. It contains no exercises, and it has few formulas saying "first do this, then do that."

This is intentional. As we'll see later, eros doesn't like to be told what to do. If you set a goal, your sexual mind will be happy to reject it. It's kind of childish and brilliant that way.

You also won't find much about sexual biology or neurochemistry on these pages. Sex books these days tend to be full of advice for "boosting your dopamine"—or your oxytocin, or some other such nonsense. In all my thirty years as a sex therapist, I've yet to see a dopamine molecule walk into my office.

We'll stick with things you can see and feel yourself, without needing a laboratory.

I'll also spare you the body diagrams. You already know what a penis and vagina look like, right? And we won't discuss how many neurons are concentrated in your clitoris. It's an impressive number, but who really cares?

There are a few great sex books already out there, and I'll point them out to you as we go along. But reading most of the others is like gnawing on dry bones. As my friend and colleague Paul Joannides, the author of *Guide to Getting It On* (one of the aforementioned great ones), has accurately noted, "the trouble with most books on sex is they don't get anyone hard or wet."

This book is not intended to get you hard or wet. But it's meant not to get in your way either. The chapters are short, so you can read them even if you get a little distracted. Hey, I *hope* you get a little distracted.

There are no lists to memorize, and there won't be a test afterward. We're dealing with a part of the human mind that hasn't gone to school yet, and never will.

Any questions?

Okay, let's get started . . .

2

The Sexual Self in Action

*Your sexual self is very honest, but its vocabulary is limited.
Usually it's limited to "yes" or "no."*

*"Go to your bosom;
Knock there, and ask your heart what it doth know . . . "*
—SHAKESPEARE, MEASURE FOR MEASURE

A young woman is in my office, telling me she doesn't feel anything during sex. Her name is Carmen. She and her husband, Scott, are recently married, and she is deeply distressed.

If you've ever not felt anything during sex with your spouse, then you know how worrying that can be. *Have I made a mistake? Do we have to get divorced? Maybe there's something wrong with him, or with me, or with us?*

It must have taken considerable courage for her to come see me. I wonder if her husband knows she's here, and what she's told him.

"I'm pretty sure there's something wrong with me sexually," she says, twirling a strand of hair around her finger.

"That's got to be a scary thought."

She nods and lets go of the strand of hair. She can't seem to find a comfortable position on my sofa.

"Is there any time you *do* feel something with him?" I try to seem as unthreatening as possible.

"Oh, yes." Big smile. Pure and open. "I love it when Scott and I kiss, on the couch in the living room," she says.

Thank God, I think to myself. *There's life here.*

She senses my relief. We both relax a little.

I try to make sure we're speaking about the same thing (always a tricky matter in this business). I ask, "When the two of you kiss, does it make you feel kind of dumb and happy? A little silly and distracted?"

"Yeah, I never thought about it, but I guess it does. I'm really pretty crazy about Scott. But then I start thinking about what's going to happen next."

"Hmm?"

"He's going to take me into the bedroom, and it's going to be a disaster. When we go into the bedroom, that's when I don't feel anything."

In Search of the Sexual Self

Many years ago two pioneers in the field of sex therapy, both medical doctors, lived on Manhattan's Upper East Side near the Cornell University School of Medicine, where they were both on the faculty.

The first, Helen Kaplan, was for a time one of the most famous sex therapists in the world. She had earned a PhD as a research psychologist before becoming a sex expert. Her book *The New Sex Therapy* became the authoritative guide to treatment for a whole generation of mental health practitioners. We'll have more to say about her later on.

The second, Avodah Offit, seemed a bit out of place in the medical field. Whereas Kaplan had trained as a scientist, Offit had originally intended to become a writer. Her work had a whimsical, philosophical style that was distinctly her own.

Offit's first book, *The Sexual Self*, was a pioneering attempt to show how sexual experience could vary according to the diversity of human character. It was widely read, and translated into several languages.

Today *The Sexual Self* is largely forgotten. Offit died in 2015, and no one ever continued her project of mapping sexual experience onto human personality.

The book's title, though, struck a note that still echoes strongly in our times. There is today a small shelf full of books whose titles include the phrase "sexual self" in some fashion—testimony to Offit's original idea that something like a sexual self existed at all.

Today the idea of a sexual self is pretty much taken for granted. But few writers on the subject have paid it much real attention, other than to recognize that it makes a catchy title.

We'll try to do better than that.

Meanwhile, Back at the Office

So far, I still don't know what the problem is with my young patient Carmen. Something is making her turn off between the living room and the bedroom. I'm pretty sure it's her sexual self trying to tell her something.

As I mentioned above, the sexual self is very honest, but its vocabulary is limited. Much of sex therapy involves trying to figure out what the sexual self, with its limited vocabulary, is actually trying to say.

Ordinarily the vocabulary of the sexual self is limited to yes or no. Getting a "no" answer in the presence of someone you've promised to spend the rest of your life with is of course very distressing.

People go to great lengths to turn a "no" into a "yes." But that's almost always a mistake. There are way better ways of handling a "no." They all involve first resolving not to freak out.

The honesty of the sexual self, like the honesty of very young children, is something we don't usually appreciate so much. We'd like the sexual self to just behave and say "yes"—so we can have the same kind of great sex everyone else is having. (Or so we think!)

But for reasons I'll get into, your sexual self tends not to listen when you tell it what to do. Like a very young child, it often has other plans entirely.

"Can you tell me what happens when you and Scott get to the bedroom?" I ask her.

"He goes inside me, and I'm wet, but I'm not really there. I'm not with him at all."

"What's wrong?"

"I don't know. He tries all different kinds of positions. He uses his hands, his mouth. And eventually he gets frustrated."

"Why? What does he want?"

"He wants me to have an orgasm."

"Do *you* want to have an orgasm?"

"Sure, if it would make him happy. But mostly I just don't want him to be so upset. It makes me feel terrible about myself—like there's something wrong with me."

Your Conditions for Good Sex

"How about when you're alone?" I ask. "Can you give yourself an orgasm then?"

"Sure. But then I have all the time in the world, and I don't have to worry about him getting upset."

I often hear this from patients—that the conditions they need for getting turned on are more easily achieved alone than with a partner. Sometimes when people get together with partners, they neglect to take responsibility for providing the conditions they need. They think their partner is supposed to get them turned on. Most people don't understand that in partner sex you're still responsible for your own turn-ons.

"How do you turn yourself on—when you're by yourself?" I ask her.

She looks down. "I don't think I'm ready to talk about that yet," she says.

Carmen studies my diplomas on the wall, taking a moment to reflect.

"Why is Scott so obsessed with giving me an orgasm?" she asks.

"I don't know," I tell her. "Maybe he just wants to do a good job."

"He thinks sex is a *job?*"

"A lot of guys do."

The question of why so many men think of sex as a job is actually a very deep one. We'll discuss it in Chapter 8. I don't mind if you skip ahead. But if you do, don't give it away, okay?

"You see the problem?" I ask. "Scott gets upset when he can't give you an orgasm. And you get upset when you can't make him happy by having one. You're feeding off each other's distress."

"Not so productive, huh?"

"Not so erotic either. It's easy to see how your sexual self might decide the situation is impossible—and just shut down."

She laughs.

Rewriting the Rules

Before Carmen leaves my office, she asks me if I have any specific advice for her.

"How about if you ask him not to try to make you climax?" I suggest.

"I could do that," she says. "Anything else?"

"How about this: You know that giddy, happy feeling you get when you're on the couch—the feeling that makes you smile?"

"Yes."

"See if you can hold on to that feeling."

"How do I do that?"

"Well, for one, maybe try staying on the couch."

Sexually we're all a bit like Pavlov's dog. Every time Pavlov fed his dog he'd ring a bell, and eventually the sound of the bell alone was enough to make the dog hungry. If the couch gives you a good

Pavlovian cue for arousal and the bed doesn't, then by all means *stay on the couch.*

I see Carmen and Scott together the next week. They sit down close together on the sofa in my office, holding hands, glancing nervously at each other and at me. After a few preliminaries, I ask Scott what Carmen told him after our last visit.

"She said you wanted us to stay on the couch." He lifts an eyebrow at me. "And for me not to try to get her to climax."

"How did that work out?"

"Well, it *was* pretty erotic having sex on the couch. Carmen seemed more into it. And she didn't get so upset afterward. But she still didn't orgasm. I guess that still bothers me."

Carmen looks up from playing with her hair. "When I was trying to climax before, it was mostly to please you," she says. She releases his hand, tucks her legs underneath her, and faces him directly on the sofa. "I don't want to do that anymore."

"I was just trying to make sure you were satisfied."

"I know. But it wasn't working. I want you to trust me that this way is much better."

"It doesn't make you frustrated?"

"What we were doing before was *way* more frustrating. Now I'm feeling close to you when we have sex. It's wonderful. I don't ever want to go back to that old way."

They're off to a good start. She's taken responsibility for her own sexual needs, and she likes how that feels. He's a bit thrown off balance by the change in her. But he also looks kind of pleased.

Is There a Wrong Way to Have an Orgasm?

The next time I see Carmen alone, she's finally ready to tell me how she climaxes when she's by herself. She stares down at her hands. "I'm pretty sure I've damaged myself somehow," she says.

"You don't seem damaged to me."

"I have orgasms the wrong way."

"*Is* there a wrong way to have an orgasm?"

"Yes," she says. And she tells me how she masturbates in the bath-tub.

It's the only way she's ever done it. Ever since she's been old enough to take baths by herself, she props up her legs and lets the running water stimulate her clitoris to orgasm. This has presented a bit of a challenge ever since she and Scott moved in together. As far as she knows, Scott has never suspected the real reason for her long baths with the door locked.

Plainly speaking, an orgasm is just a reflex. But we humans never experience anything plainly. Everything has meaning. If every time you give yourself an orgasm you feel you're doing it the wrong way, then over the years this idea will gather a lot of power. And the likelihood of your feeling relaxed and excited enough to have an orgasm with someone you love will be slim.

All good psychotherapies are based on acceptance. This is even more true in sex therapy.

Acceptance is "vitamin A" for sex. Your sexual self is never going to be happy unless you feel accepted in bed for who you are. And if your sexual self isn't happy, nobody's going to be happy.

You'll find information about how to get more vitamin A in just about every chapter of this book. For now, let's just say that if you need to use running water to have an orgasm, that's just fine.

But there is a kind of magic that occurs when a person who's never used their own hands for sexual excitement starts to do that for the first time. After many weeks Carmen decides to try using her hands to give herself an orgasm, and the experience convinces her she's neither broken nor damaged. At that point she has nothing more to dread or to prove.

I see Carmen and Scott one last time together, and they are quite changed. Now they look like people who are having good sex: giggly and alive, in that ridiculously effervescent way that good sex should make you look.

Carmen tells me that now she's able to hold on to feeling aroused as long as she wants when she and Scott are together—even in the bedroom. She hasn't had an orgasm yet with him inside her. But she's given herself plenty of them in his arms.

I'm not particularly worried. It's more important whether you're genuinely aroused than where and how you climax.

Your sexual self is very honest. Trust what it tells you, and it will usually teach you what you need to know.

Your True Colors

In 1989 when I was just starting out as a sex therapist, another young woman came to see me deeply distressed about her marriage. Sarina had been having sex with her husband one evening and she'd started to cry and hadn't been able to stop.

I asked her what was wrong. She said it wasn't any one thing in particular. Everything worked fine, but for some reason the experience didn't touch her. She didn't feel anything special.

"Do you love your husband?" I asked.

"Yes, but there's something missing."

"Something about the sex?"

"Maybe." Sarina looked uncertain, and cried a little more. "No, the sex is okay. But there's something else I need, that I'm not getting."

"Tell me about it."

"I don't know. It's a feeling of 'Yes, that's me.'"

"Have you ever felt that with anyone?" I asked.

"Yes, in college. But it was with a woman."

"Were you in love with her?"

"Yes."

And so began Sarina's journey to find out who she really was. Even though the American Psychiatric Association had decided much earlier, in 1973, that homosexuality was not a disease, I still had gay people coming to see me in 1989 asking if I knew how to cure them of it.

I had no idea how to do that, of course. And neither did anyone else, because it can't be done. If you have a strong same-sex attraction, it's just a part of who you are. The question is how thoroughly you (and the people around you) are able to accept it.

Sarina ended up divorcing her husband. And after much searching she ended up happily partnered with a woman, with whom she raised two children. She came to see me again several times for various other reasons, which I'll tell you about later. But I still often think back to the time we first met in 1989, when I first started to ponder the relationship between sexuality and the self.

Most heterosexual people don't have to spend so much time figuring out what they really feel—or who they really are. If you're straight, all you have to do is swim with the prevailing current.

These days, even if you're exclusively or predominantly gay or lesbian, that's relatively easier to figure out. You have more good role models. Ordeals like the kind Sarina went through as a young woman are less common now. In many parts of this country, most gay and lesbian young people's sexual identities are now fully formed by the end of high school.

But there are still young adults in traditional or religious communities today whose journeys closely parallel the one Sarina took in 1989.

What's more, some people have sexual and gender variations that still haven't yet been fully understood or accepted by the larger culture. If you're bisexual, transgender, or just very kinky, you're still likely to have to craft your own sexual identity as you go along. That's an extraordinarily difficult thing to do.

People who are bisexual have historically been seen as not really belonging to either the straight or gay communities. But recently there's been a big jump in people self-identifying as bisexual, so that's likely to change.

We humans are so sexually diverse that a catalog of all our diversity would be limited only by the number of categories we could imagine. Some young people these days prefer newer and less restrictive categories, such as "mostly straight" or "heteroflexible." And some have thrown away categories completely, in favor of just "queer."

When it comes to eros, we all have a need to express our true colors. It's not just about the sex. It's often about love too. As Joe Kort and Alexander Morgan emphasize in their book *Is My Husband Gay, Straight, or Bi?*, it's less about whom you want to go to bed with and more about whom you want to wake up with.

Most of all it's about who you are. There's something uniquely validating about an erotic relationship where you feel, "Yes, that's me."

Sex and Human Feelings

It's not immediately clear why sex should be such an emotional thing for people. There is no other human appetite that we obsess so much about—or that arouses such strong feelings. Why should sex have such power to make us feel so wonderful—or so terrible—about ourselves?

To answer that question, we'll need to understand more about where sexual feelings get their start. The answer will make it very clear why sex is so emotional, why it involves the self at all, and why we're all of us so terribly vulnerable in bed.

Let's take a look.

3

Be My Baby

Your sexual self never grows up.
No matter how old you are, it remains a small child.

"We live to be touched."
—AVODAH OFFIT, *THE SEXUAL SELF*

A Hot and Humid August Day

A few years ago, the following fragment made the rounds of various
sex therapy internet lists. Its source and author are uncertain:

It was a hot and humid August day, and
they had been perspiring. Now it was dusk.
The apartment was empty save for the two of
them. As they lay in warm embrace, this room,
this bed, was the universe. Aside from the faint sounds of
their tranquil breathing, they were silent. She stroked the
nape of his neck. He nuzzled her erect nipple, first gently
with his nose—then licked it, tasted, smelled and absorbed
her scent. He pressed his body close to hers, sighed, and
fully spent, closed his eyes and soon fell into a deep
satisfying sleep. Ever so slowly she slipped herself out
from under him, lest she disturb him, cradled him in her arms,
and moved him to his crib.

The best lovemaking often looks a lot like mother-infant bonding. All that holding, stroking, and eye gazing. Those satisfied, dreamy, out-of-focus smiles on both your faces.

Did you ever wonder why so many love songs have the word "baby"? Now you know.

Eros recalls our attachment to the first people who held us, rocked us, enjoyed us, and told us we were wonderful. Sex is one area of life where it's okay, even desirable, for adults to feel a bit childlike. When lovemaking is at its best, you feel in touch with your deepest, most valuable self.

As sex therapists we do our best to help people get aroused, have good orgasms, and so on. But what we *really* want is for them to laugh, and giggle, and be silly and selfish and vulnerable, and to enjoy the kind of total absorption that as an adult you only really get when you're having sex.

Once you understand that eros is infantile, it's easy to see why sex is such an emotional thing for people. And why few things can make you feel quite as good about yourself. Or quite as bad.

The Joy of Sex

> *During sex, the main thing is to enjoy your partner*
> *and feel they're enjoying you.*
> *Everything else is secondary.*

To enjoy and be enjoyed is the essence of good lovemaking. No doubt this too goes back to childhood.

Children need desperately to be enjoyed. A mother examining her baby's feet may feel grateful that they are healthy and normal. She may want to memorize the look and feel of them, knowing that they will change so much in the years to come. It's essential though that she also enjoy them. Later in her child's life it may make a big difference for her son or daughter to remember, in whatever vague unconscious way, that someone long ago felt joy simply because he or she existed.

I spend a lot of time talking with people who just don't feel their partners enjoy them anymore. It always makes me sad.

Years ago, a middle-aged man who'd come to see me about his not-very-sexual marriage struck up an email correspondence with a woman he'd met at an office function. Every time he received an email from her, he would get an erection. There was something about this new woman's obvious pleasure in writing him that touched his sexual soul in a way it hadn't been touched for years.

Many other men would have seen this as a sign that they were married to the wrong woman. But he was sensible enough to conclude that he had simply fallen off his proper path. With a little coaching, he and his wife easily found their way back. She was just as relieved as he to feel enjoyed again.

When I was in training, often one of the first questions I'd be asked about a new patient was "Do you like the patient?" It struck me as a silly question at the time, but now I recognize it as an important one. Patients need to be enjoyed too. If you really like them, they're much more likely to get better.

Of Sweaty T-Shirts and the Tops of Babies' Heads

Scent is the perfect expression of eros. You can't hold it, touch it, eat it, or do anything with it but enjoy it. Scent is the most intimate form of connection—experienced only at very close range—and the last threshold before full-on physical intimacy.

Scent and desire share common quarters. The top of a baby's head has a fragrance as powerful as the most aromatic flower. The scent of a mother's breast must be equally intoxicating to a nursing infant. It's likely that every baby feels their mother's scent is perfect, and that this perfection forms the template for all future erotic experiences.

I discovered many years ago that if you ask the happiest couples what keeps them together, very often the answer is "We like the way each other smells." It's no accident that single people talk about finding someone with the right "chemistry."

My patients who are actively dating tease me sometimes for being so curious about how their dates smell. I worry a bit when a woman tells me she doesn't want to get close to her new boyfriend until he's had a shower. I look forward to the day when she finds someone and can't wait to bury her face in his sweat-soaked T-shirt.

Fragrance designers know how to arrange scents to correspond to a typical night's seduction. The scents one first notices on a date are known as the "top notes"—or, for short, "the top."

Often fruity and sweet, they bring a quick smile of pleasure. But these are really just fancy wrapping for the more valuable package inside. It's only later, over dinner perhaps, that you experience the "heart"—the heavier scents. And much later that the heaviest scents, the "base," begin to stir as clothes come off in preparation for lovemaking.

When you were very young, physical sensation and emotion were all wrapped together in one package. During lovemaking, they still are. Really good sex evokes infancy in all its contradictory aspects—tender yet ruthless, urgent yet relaxed, serious and carefree at the same time. If all goes well, at the moment of orgasm you become an infant pulling at the breast for dear life—then afterward finally giving in to drowsiness, like a small child falling asleep on its mother's lap.

A Baby on the Train

A long time ago, a young woman patient of mine was having an unhappy love affair and wanted to end it but for some reason could not. The self she experienced with her lover was not her usual self. Ordinarily confident and expressive, in his presence she would be passive and sullen.

Before long, she began having vivid memories of having been molested as a young girl. Spend some time with someone who has been sexually abused, and you will never again doubt for a moment that sex and the self are inextricably bound.

Most survivors of sexual abuse instinctively feel that their sexuality is not truly their own. For this young woman, sex was something she did for other people. The person she became during the act seemed to be a remnant of the frightened, angry child she had once been—a kind of memory really, but never fully realized or expressed in words.

To replace a fragmentary form of memory like this with a fuller recollection of facts and feelings is one of the most fundamental activities of psychotherapy. As my patient began to accomplish this, she began to take ownership of her body and her arousal in a new way.

She came in one day and told me she'd dreamed she was on a train, nursing a newborn. (Trains and other forms of transportation in dreams often refer to therapy itself.) The baby had begun to turn cold and to freeze solid. She felt terrified. But then the baby thawed, and came back to life, healthy and pink.

Waking up, she felt she immediately knew what the baby in the dream signified. In her words: "It's my sexuality. It's mine. It's me."

Your sexual self can't hide its feelings, and it can't pretend. That's its crowning glory: to be infantile, in the best sense of the word. That's where we all start from, and in bed that's who we still are.

The Egotism of Toddlers

On the infantile level, sex is pretty simple. Infants haven't developed much of an ego yet. They don't seem to require self-affirmation in the ordinary adult sense. They don't experience pride, shame, envy, or self-doubt.

Those feelings arrive with a bang in your second year of life. By the time you're a toddler, your need for self-affirmation has become enormous. This poses all sorts of challenges, and lays the groundwork for most of the problems of adult erotic life.

Good lovemaking has a serious quality to it. Sex may be blissful at times, but it is never exactly festive, or amusing. It's a serious kind of fun.

We adults don't just want sex to feel good. We want sex to make us feel good about ourselves. There tends to be a certain amount of pride involved. When sex goes well, we feel deeply validated. When it doesn't, we can feel devastated.

This connection between sex and self-regard is the main thing that keeps us sex therapists in business.

The Other Side of Saturday Night

Sunday mornings I usually go to the office for a few hours—to escape the noise of my kids watching TV at home, to catch up on some paperwork, and to enjoy the peace and quiet. One spring Sunday morning I get to the office to find a message from a young man named Paul, saying he needs to speak to me right away.

A message like this on a Sunday morning almost always means someone lost an erection Saturday night.

Not particularly wanting to face the pile of paperwork on my desk, I decide to call him. He sounds surprised to hear back from me so early on a Sunday morning.

No one knows exactly why losing an erection is such a horrible experience for a man. All we know for sure is that young men who lose their erections are desperate people.

"Is there any chance I could see you today?" he asks. I make myself a dubious promise to take care of my paperwork tomorrow, and I tell him to come on over.

Paul rings my buzzer a half hour later, sits down in my waiting room and exhales deeply.

"Thanks so much, man," he says. He's a tall, handsome young person in his late twenties with a firm handshake and a broad smile, wearing a rumpled polo shirt and khaki shorts. I find out he's an investment banker from the Midwest living with roommates somewhere in Tribeca.

He's obviously had a very sleepless night. Some of it, I assume, Googling "sex therapist NYC" online. He very much needs a shave.

Paul looks around my office, fidgets a bit in his chair, then proceeds to tell me the story of what happened the night before on a date with a woman whom he says he's very interested in.

It was their third date, which is usually a big deal in Manhattan. If a single woman in New York has agreed to a third date, there's a good chance she's interested in having sex.

Last night was no exception. After a delicious meal, a few glasses of wine, and some slow dancing to music at a club downtown, she took him back to her apartment and they started to undress. He felt very excited. But to his surprise a few minutes later when she wanted him inside her, suddenly he had no erection at all. Zero.

She tried every way she could to make him hard again, but each time the result was the same. Zero. Nothing. She was very nice about it and said it was okay. But it was the most miserable night of his life.

What had gone wrong?

Simple. To paraphrase our first "rule" from Chapter 2, "Your sexual organs are very honest, but their vocabulary is limited to 'yes' or 'no.'" Clearly his penis just decided to say "no" in the only language it had.

But why "no" with this particular woman, on this particular Saturday night? You can't always be sure. It could be anything, really. Often a woman will assume it's just because he didn't like her body very much once he got her naked. But the real reasons are usually emotional rather than sexual.

I ask Paul to go through the story again. "You're positive you were attracted to her?" I ask.

"No question," he says. "I was so hard when we were dancing together that it was actually a little embarrassing."

"And later, when the two of you got undressed?"

"About as turned on as I've ever been. I put on a condom, no problem. But then just at the crucial moment, when everything was going so well, I lost it. Zero."

"Any idea why?"

"Not a clue."

Paradoxical, right? A man gets hard with a woman on the dance floor, then loses his erection when she offers him her willing vagina. Go figure.

Popular opinion tends to attribute such a thing to "performance anxiety." But this has never made much sense to me. Why should intercourse be more of a performance than anything else?

"Before you lost it, were you feeling anxious?" I ask him.

"Not really. Just very excited."

Sometimes it's some other negative emotion. I run through the usual possibilities. Guilt? Resentment? Grief? I don't find much to work with.

Maybe he had a really messed up childhood? No, everything seems to have been fine there.

Then it occurs to me:

Maybe the problem is that he's developed feelings for this woman.

"Tell me about her," I say to Paul. "You like her a lot?"

"Actually, I think I'm in love with her."

That's noteworthy. Handsome young bankers in Manhattan typically go through a lot of beautiful women, rarely falling in love with any of them. I wonder what it is about this one that's attracted him so powerfully.

"Have you told her how you feel about her?"

"No, it was just our third date. I figure I'll see whether it lasts, before I tell her."

"Does she feel the same way about you?"

"I think so. At least I hope so—after last night!"

Most women will give a man a pass if he loses his erection the first couple of times in bed. They know that men are ordinarily somewhat challenged in the intimate realm.

Most heterosexual boys feel the need to escape their mother's embrace in order to become men. The love of a grown woman is a return to something that a man may have given up years ago with great difficulty.

To feel deeply about a new woman can be a little frightening, and his sexual self may react accordingly. I've known many men who can function perfectly well with a partner, unless they've fallen in love with her.

One of the paradoxes of human intimate life is that we tend to fall in love with relative strangers. We're less likely to be stirred to passion by people we've known since kindergarten, and more likely to lust after someone we've just met. This can pose a problem for the sexual self—which like a small child always yearns for the familiar.

No child wants to be handed over to a total stranger. I'm convinced that when a new erotic relationship works well, it's because there are enough signs of familiarity that this new person doesn't really feel so new. I'm sure you've felt that sense of instant closeness with a stranger from time to time, right?

With sex it's different though. In bed it's physically obvious that this person is new—that you don't really know them at all.

"Look," I tell him, "the first thing you should know is that your penis is working fine. It's just saying 'no' at the moment, which is what it's built to do when things don't feel quite right."

He looks worried. "You think my penis doesn't like her?"

"No, just the opposite. I think it likes her a little too much at the moment. I think you might be worried about getting hurt."

"So what should I do?"

"You want a suggestion? Next time you get together, tell her you're very attracted to her but you need to know her a little better first. Maybe just relax in bed together for a little while, without having sex."

"Won't that make her feel frustrated?"

"Maybe a little. But she'll like that you're telling her what's going on. Women tend to get exhausted trying to guess. They usually appreciate any information you can give them."

Paul gives this some thought. "Okay, but what if I get excited?"

"Just enjoy it."

"I don't know what you mean."

"It's good to be excited. Just enjoy it."

"And not jump on her?"

"Not just yet. Not until you know her a little better. For now, just *enjoy* her. That's going to be the royal road to your getting better."

"How about Viagra?"

"Well, it's a judgment call. Most cases of 'shy penis' like yours get better within a couple of weeks. But if you want to have a backup, then sure. It's just sometimes tricky to get off the medication. Viagra doesn't cause physical dependence, but you can start to feel naked without it."

He says he'll take a prescription from me, just to be on the safe side.

I don't hear from him again. But a few weeks later I think I see him at a restaurant in the neighborhood, having dinner with an exceptionally beautiful young woman. I can't help but be curious about the state of his erections.

From the way she's smiling and leaning into him, I'd guess things are going well. But hey, you never know.

~~

A year later, Paul comes to see me again. He looks much better with a shave. He and the very beautiful woman are living together now. She wants to get married. He's thinking about it and wants to talk things over with me.

Sure, I tell him. But first I'm curious what ended up happening with his erections.

"Oh, that," he says, smiling. "It was funny. I didn't tell you back then, but when I met her last year she'd recently broken up with someone else—someone who has a pretty big name in my business. I think I was in awe of her—and of *him*, though I didn't realize it at the time. You know what I mean?"

"Actually that's a pretty common reason guys lose erections. You get psyched out by the competition. I'm sorry I didn't ask about that as a possibility."

"You know what finally did the trick?" he says. "One night I asked her point-blank: 'Why do you want me, when you could have *him*?' It felt like a lame thing to ask, but I realized that was the question that had been on my mind from the start."

"What'd she *say*?"

"She smiled, and said I didn't have anything to worry about. She and the other guy hadn't been very happy together. She told me I made her feel happy like a little girl again, and that she loved me very much."

"Nice."

"And here's what's funny. Right away, I got hard and we had sex. But to tell you the truth, the sex didn't feel as significant as just finding out that she really wanted me."

"Did she tell you anything else?" I ask.

"Actually, yes. She said she liked the way I smelled."

~~~

A man instinctively remembers having been the object of his mother's exclusive attention. Somewhere within him he can still recall feeling her joy in his small body, his scent, his being. But that was long ago, before he learned you need to compete with other men who might have an edge on you.

A man will usually choose someone who makes him feel he doesn't have to compete so hard for their love. Someone who enjoys him just as he is.

But he'll likely keep his eyes open—just in case.

4

Selfishly Yours

Your sexual self doesn't just want to be loved.
It wants to be loved more than anyone or anything
in the world.

"Being chosen by the one you chose is one of the glories of fall-
ing in love. It generates a feeling of intense personal importance."
—ESTHER PEREL, *MATING IN CAPTIVITY*

Quick, what's a two-year-old's favorite word?

You know the answer, of course: "Mine."

We humans are a possessive bunch. It's no accident that those little candy hearts we give each other on Valentine's Day say "Be Mine."

In whatever language, the word "mine" has long been a favorite with lovers all over the world—probably since the dawn of human pair-bonding.

You know that famous verse from the Bible? *"I am my beloved's, and my beloved is mine."*

Who talks like that?

Two-year-olds, of course. And lovers. It's in our nature.

We humans work hard to control our possessive instincts. We spend years teaching our young children not to be so grabby. But when it comes to erotic life, that all goes out the window.

Growing up, we all come to learn that we're not the center of the universe, and that the people who love us also have other concerns. But eros is primitive, and the erotic mind is a poor student. Your sexual self retains from infancy an image of pure, absolute attention from an adoring other.

Basically, it just wants to be worshipped.

Your Inner Narcissist

Wait a minute, you say. The sexual self is sounding pretty narcissistic.

Yes, and that's as it should be.

Let me explain—

You're probably accustomed to thinking of "narcissism" as something negative. That's *pathological* narcissism: when people need constant praise and don't really care about anyone else.

Healthy narcissism is different. It's what keeps you looking out for your own best interests in life. Without it, people would walk all over you, and you'd let them.

You probably know some individuals who don't have enough healthy narcissism. It's not pretty, is it?

Infants and toddlers are little fountains of healthy narcissism. They're honest and direct about what they need, and they have the energy to insist on it if they don't get it. Young children never worry about whether their needs might be excessive. They just want what they want.

As the years go by, the generous amount of healthy narcissism that you started with as a child gradually gets depleted as you meet with disappointments in life. That's normal. It's the essence of growing up.

If you're lucky, the disappointments aren't too severe. One of a parent's principal jobs is to trim your child's healthy narcissism without destroying it. No, you can't have your mother's attention all the time. But if you behave yourself she'll read you a story before she puts you to bed.

Bit by bit, the grandiosity of early childhood gets replaced by something more practical. No, you'll never be a movie star or play professional football. But work hard and follow the rules, and you'll probably do okay.

Your sexual self resists being tamed in this way. No matter how grown up you get, your sexual self remains saturated with the ridiculously expansive narcissism of childhood. You may be a model of humility outside the bedroom. But in bed you'll still want to be fussed over and adored and treated like the most important person in the world.

That's just the way it is.

The Passion Prescription

Healthy narcissism gives the erotic mind its energy and vitality. A certain kind of selfishness is an advantage in lovemaking. We ordinarily refer to it as "passion."

> *Sexual selfishness tends to be more erotic than sexual generosity. Being a generous lover isn't a bad thing of course. But if it's not accompanied by the right kind of selfishness then it can be a problem.*

A man comes to see me for advice on how to please his wife in bed. He says her needs are very particular. For instance, the two of them will be involved in some kind of foreplay, and she'll interrupt him with criticisms like "Stop, that's too much," or "No, not like that."

The poor man tries his best to please her, or at least not to upset her. But the harder he tries, the more frustrated she gets.

He's at his wit's end.

Fortunately I know this story well, having heard it so many times over the years from so many men. When I first started as a sex therapist, I'd routinely ask to speak with the wife in private, and here's how the conversation usually went:

Dr. S: *Your husband says he doesn't know how to please you. He says you're very sensitive.*

Wife: *Oh, for heaven's sake—I'm not sensitive at all. I'm just dying inside for him to show me a little passion. All he does is fumble around. It drives me crazy.*

You see the problem, right?

He's focused on trying to satisfy *her*. But all she really wants is to feel *his* passion, *his* confidence, *his* hunger to devour her in an ecstasy of selfish abandon. She wants to feel his healthy narcissism directed at her.

But by this point in the relationship he doesn't have much healthy narcissism left. How could he, with all the criticism she's leveled at him over the years?

There's a simple solution to this dilemma. It begins with asking the question "What's more erotic, a partner who just wants to give you sexual pleasure, or a partner who wants to *take* sexual pleasure from being with you?"

The answer is obvious, right? Sexual generosity that's not accompanied by a certain kind of selfishness just isn't very erotic. No hero in a romance novel ever rips off the heroine's clothes and says, "Now tell me how you like to be touched."

Most people, men and women alike, prefer lovers whose absorption in the moment makes them at least momentarily "thoughtless." Most of us quite enjoy being hungrily devoured by someone we love. Assuming they properly relish us first.

Power Play

Power is the ultimate aphrodisiac.
—HENRY KISSINGER

The sexual self loves power. Of course it does. It's a child.

Children tend to be highly attracted to power. Adults are attracted to power too, but with children it's more obvious.

Fireworks, for example, are a highly concentrated form of power. Most children love everything about fireworks. The sudden splash of bright color, the smoke, the absurdly loud noise. The audible gasp of surprise from the crowd.

We adults tend to enjoy fireworks as well. But that's because they take us back to the thrill of raw power that we felt as children. It's always more fun to see fireworks in the company of a child.

Eros lives at the border between safety and adventure. Safety anchors it. Nothing works in bed if you don't feel safe. (Okay, unless you are *really* kinky.) But safety alone won't do it. Most of us need a bit of power play in bed as well.

No, I'm not talking about bondage. (Though I have nothing against bondage, if that's what gets you going.) I mean something more general: the ordinary exchange of power that accompanies good lovemaking.

Many people's favorite part of sex is that moment when the other person kind of loses control just as they're about to have an orgasm. The louder their cries of passion, the better. People cherish that feeling of power they get when their partner has a really impressive climax.

Power play is at the root of most sexual fantasies. Arousal without fantasy tends to produce feelings of pleasure and gratitude. Add fantasy, and the experience will likely involve some feeling of *triumph* as well.

Nancy Friday's 1973 collection of women's sexual fantasies, *My Secret Garden*, contains many fantasies where the triumph is overt, and many where it's more or less concealed. In one, a young woman imagines that her mother is presenting her at the court of a powerful rajah. The young woman keeps her gaze fixed downward as her mother undresses her and points out in great detail to the entire court how exquisite her daughter's body is.

Watching this demonstration, the rajah and his court all become intensely aroused.

A traditionally masculine form of power encounters a classically feminine form of it, and the result is a rocking good party for all concerned.

The original account in *My Secret Garden* is much more explicit. But you get the idea.

Jill

With some fantasies—especially the more kinky ones—you have to use your imagination to find the narcissistic triumph hidden deep in the story.

Jill came across the park from the Upper East Side this morning to see me. Her husband, Peter, does something with real estate, and she takes care of their two young children full-time at home.

Jill says she's very attracted to Peter. She gets excited and she always has an orgasm. But she finds the whole thing upsetting. I try my best to figure out what the problem is, but by the end of her first visit I still don't have a clue.

Today is our second appointment, and Jill is wearing a determined expression that I know must mean something. She gets to it right away:

"There's something I haven't told you yet," she says. "I have a fantasy that I use when I want to climax. I hate it, but it's the only thing that works."

She looks away and studies the books on my shelf.

"Would it be okay for you to tell me what the fantasy is?" I ask.

"No, not really!" She laughs nervously. "But I figure if I don't, then it's not much use coming here to see you." She takes a deep breath.

"I imagine a very wicked man has captured me and locked me up somewhere. I can't see him, but I can feel his eyes on me and I know he wants me."

"When you imagine this, it helps you climax?"

"Every time."

She looks away, embarrassed.

"Any idea what this fantasy is about?" I ask her.

"I don't really want to know," she says. She looks down, measuring her words carefully as she adjusts her skirt. "I just want you to help me get rid of it, so I can have an orgasm the normal way like everyone else."

She waits expectantly, as I try to figure out how to respond.

I'm not sure I can give her what she wants. The truth is, you can't just get rid of sexual fantasies. It's usually a bad idea to even try.

I want to tell her, "Look, this fantasy may have a story behind it that needs to be heard and understood." But I resist the impulse. She's not looking to understand anything. She just wants to have an orgasm "the normal way."

I want to give her a lecture about the word "normal," and how troublesome it can be for people. But the stern look on her face makes it clear that this too would be a waste of time.

Trying hard to come up with something helpful, I review what she's told me so far:

In the fantasy, someone has locked Jill up. She can't see him, but she knows he's getting very excited watching her. What's this all about?

Well for one, it has danger in it, which turns a lot of people on. Anyone who's spent an hour watching HBO knows that danger can be sexy. We're all profoundly attracted to lust and aggression—

especially when they're combined together. (If you have any doubt, just watch *Game of Thrones*.)

Then there's the power aspect—which as I mentioned is pretty much a universal in sex fantasies. A lot of women fantasize during sex about being powerless, but that's just the surface layer. Deeper down, the reverse is also usually true.

In Jill's fantasy, the man has total power over her. But she has total power over him too, since he can't take his eyes off her irresistible body. A good fantasy will get you coming and going like that.

Might any of this help Jill feel better right now? Not likely. I sense anxiety turning to frustration within her, as I struggle to come up with something helpful to say.

Then something occurs to me:

This fantasy is all about *attention*. Jill's captor may be wicked, but he's clearly giving her a whole basketful of attention.

Lust can sometimes come in handy when you really want to be noticed.

Not all kinky fantasies contain stories. Some people just seem to be kinky from birth. Their kinky turn-ons are simply part of who they are, just like anyone else's more ordinary erotic preferences. Nothing to explain. But this particular recurrent kinky fantasy of Jill's feels as if it's trying to tell a story. I'd like to know what the story is.

You have to be careful though. Intense, repetitive fantasies can be a form of memory, and the memories involved are usually very painful. One of the most important functions of fantasy is to soothe trauma by sweetening it with sexual pleasure. Sex and sadness don't sit very well together.

Was Jill abandoned when she was young? In her fantasy she's alone, scared, and turned on. I wonder if originally she was just alone and scared.

Genders switch around in fantasies sometimes, just like in dreams. The unseen person who can't take his eyes off her seems like something a child might wish if her mother was far away: You can't see her, but you know she's always there, watching you.

"When you were young, did you ever really need someone's attention but couldn't get it?" I ask her.

"Why?"

"Your fantasy. It seems like it's all about having someone's complete attention."

Jill's expression changes to something softer. "Funny you should mention that," she says. "My mother was very young when she had me. Too young. She used to leave me with the neighbors a lot. I remember waiting and waiting for her to come home."

"Do you remember how you felt when she got home?"

"Confused. Relieved, but angry. Sometimes I wouldn't talk to her for hours afterward."

So much emotion. So sad. We therapists always arrive on the scene a few decades too late.

"Why are you asking me this?" she asks.

Should I tell her? I'm not sure. I've opened the door, but I don't know if the time is right yet to walk her through it.

In the end, I decide that telling her will probably be more useful than not telling her.

"I think your fantasy contains a memory of feeling abandoned by your mother," I say. "In the fantasy you're anxious and alone, just like it happened in real life. But the fantasy does something else—something wonderful, really. It puts somebody there to keep you company. You can't see him, but he's always watching you."

I scan Jill's face. She looks attentive, interested, a bit surprised.

Then a moment of confusion. "If it's really my mother," she asks, "then why is it a *man*?"

"I don't know. Fantasies switch gender sometimes. The fact that you know it's a man probably gives the fantasy a more powerful erotic buzz. It might also help disguise the real situation."

"Weird," she says.

"Yes, but it kind of makes sense to me."

"To me too, actually."

"Good. I know you hate this fantasy, but I'm hoping someday you might actually come to appreciate it. It's kind of creative, in its own way."

"I have to think about this," she says, looking away. Her fingers quietly drum on the arm of her chair.

"Look," she says, turning to face me again. "I don't think this fantasy is ever going to give me much pleasure. There's just too much hostility in it. Just once I'd like to climax with Peter while thinking about something *happy*. Isn't there any way to do that?"

Now that she's put it that way, it seems like a fair request. After all, this is *sex therapy*. It's *supposed* to be about happy. And she's been a champ so far, putting up with all these interpretations of mine. The least I can do is to help her find a more agreeable way to have an orgasm.

"Here's something you might try," I tell her. "The next time you have sex with Peter, pay careful attention to the details. What exactly are you feeling? What else is going on? Be objective, like a reporter. Let's get all the information."

"That'll help me get rid of it?"

"If you still want to. But first let's get all the facts."

Shame

Jill and I make an appointment for the following week. I worry about how she's going to react to all the information I've given her today. Sometimes despite my best efforts to be encouraging, someone will take something I said or did and use it to prove that I think they're hopeless.

Why? Usually because they're overburdened with shame.

We mental health practitioners think of shame the way dental hygienists think of plaque. Everybody gets it, some more than others, but if you let it get out of hand it can cause you all sorts of problems.

It's important to distinguish between shame and guilt, since we humans are so vulnerable to both. Guilt means feeling bad about something you've *done* (or thought of doing). It's painful, but useful. Feeling guilty makes you to want to confess, or make it right, or not do it in the first place. Without guilt, we'd all be sociopaths.

Shame is another matter entirely. Whereas guilt says you *did* something bad, shame says you *are* bad. Guilt makes you want to atone. Shame makes you want to run and hide, so no one will see you.

For some reason shame and sexuality seem to go together. According to Genesis, Adam and Eve first experience shame after eating from the fruit of the Tree of Knowledge. They make themselves clothes because they realize they're naked.

No one actually knows why human beings first started covering themselves up. The Bible says it was because they felt shame. But the reverse can also be true: Once you start to cover something up, it's natural to feel ashamed of it. As they say in the twelve-step programs, "You're only as sick as your secrets."

I'm aware that Jill has never spoken aloud to another human being the things she's told me. It's a serious responsibility, and one I don't take lightly.

I'm glad she came to see me instead of someone who doesn't hear about sex all day. Since I'm a sex therapist, I've heard so many curious fantasies from perfectly normal people that I no longer react much to them. It's often a relief to my patients that I don't think the details of their erotic lives are that remarkable.

~

When I first started out as a sex therapist, the rule was that you had to be part of a couple to be in treatment. Sex therapy was by definition a kind of couple's therapy.

This never made much sense to me. Sure, some couples are so knotted up emotionally that you really have to see them together. But often it's more productive to see someone alone. Once they figure out what they need and how to ask for it, the problem may be solved.

Sex is fundamentally selfish. To connect through mutual selfishness may well be the root source of all erotic blessings. You may care deeply about your partner, but at peak arousal it's nice if you can take them momentarily for granted.

That's paradoxical, of course. But when has sex ever *not* been paradoxical?

You may be a gentle, reasonable person in the rest of your life, but during good lovemaking it's best if at times you can let yourself feel momentarily drunk with power.

To have good sex with someone you love, it can sometimes be important to love them a little less—to become momentarily oblivious to their needs and trust them to take care of themselves.

The Art of the Easy

Life is difficult. Sex should be easy.
If it's not easy, then you're not doing it right.

"It's natural for humans to seek out joy and pleasure.
We're born that way and then get talked out of it."
—CHRISTIANE NORTHRUP, M.D.
WOMEN'S BODIES, WOMEN'S WISDOM

The essence of good foreplay is to enjoy yourself.

Sounds obvious, huh? You'd be surprised.

A lot of people think foreplay is just to supply a woman with enough physical stimulation. I see hundreds of couples in my office where the man thinks the main goal is to get his partner wet.

Most sex books certainly don't help. A lot of them go on and on about how you need to "pleasure your partner." Boring, boring, boring.

The unfortunate thing about these sex books is that people read them. The result is an endless parade of men in my office who try to pleasure their partners just right and end up boring them to tears.

Of course it's important to remember what your wife likes and doesn't like in bed. But simply knowing how to give her pleasure is not enough.

She also needs to know that her body is giving *you* pleasure.

Does Fingering Work?

> *It is not uncommon for me to get a random text from my kids'*
> *teenaged friends inquiring about sexual issues . . . One text that made*
> *me laugh out loud recently asked, "Does fingering even work???"*
> —WENDY STRGAR, "FOREPLAY'S HARVEST"

No, fingering doesn't "work." The structure of the question is wrong from the start.

If stroking your partner's vulva with your fingers excites both of you, then I'm all for it. But if it feels like work, stop right away.

Don't do it just to get her off. Sooner or later, she'll realize there's no passion in it.

The same goes for oral sex.

I'm fundamentally opposed to the idea of "giving oral sex." During oral sex, you should be *taking* too—not just giving.

My colleague Ian Kerner wrote a wonderful book called *She Comes First* about how to give a woman great cunnilingus. *She Comes First* has the best cunnilingus techniques in the world. But these techniques are only really useful if cunnilingus is something you like to do.

Some straight men, for example, just love everything about the vulva—its warmth, its wetness, its scent. Others are neutral about it. And some, even after extensive counseling, say getting up close to their partner's vulva is just not their thing—even though she may turn them on in every other way.

It's the same with fellatio. Some people just love taking their partner's penis in their mouth. Some don't really have much feeling about it either way. Others don't like it at all.

Whether it's oral sex, fingering, or even intercourse, here's the bottom line: Unless you genuinely like doing it, soon or later it's going to feel like work.

Sex should never feel like work. If it feels like work, stop immediately.

Don't just do it because you like to hear your partner moan. Go find something else that makes them moan that you actually enjoy.

Jill's Next Appointment

I mentally prepare for the hour of Jill's next appointment, and I imagine her doing the same. When I come out to the waiting room, she turns away slightly. This must be a little embarrassing.

"How did it go with Peter this week?" I ask.

"Well, I did what you said. I took detailed mental notes."

"Did you discover anything new?"

"No, just the usual. We had sex, I got excited. Then just as I was about to have an orgasm, I lost it like I always do."

"That suddenly? Right at the last minute?" I don't remember her telling me that before.

"Absolutely. Gone. That's when I use the fantasy. It's the only way I can get off."

No wonder she feels so frustrated.

"You know, this is really important information," I tell her. "Trying to have an orgasm when you're no longer really turned on isn't going to make you feel good. Kinky or not."

"I shouldn't try to have an orgasm?"

"Not if you're not turned on. That's too much work."

"But it feels so terrible to lose arousal like that."

No, I think to myself. *Loss of arousal doesn't by itself feel terrible. Frustrating, certainly. Disappointing, without question. But "terrible" is one of those over-the-top words that to a therapist signals we're dealing with something else.*

"Why do you think it feels so terrible?" I ask.

She rolls her eyes and gives me an exasperated look. "What part of not being able to have an orgasm don't you understand?"

"I think the worst part must be what it *means* to you."

"You mean that I'm all messed up?"

"Sure. How erotic is that?"

She smiles sadly. "But what if it's true?" she asks.

"Why don't you find out for yourself?"

"What do you mean?"

"Try not working so hard at it, and see what happens. Sex shouldn't be such hard work. Maybe that will help."

"But what if I lose my arousal?"

"Easy. Just hit 'rewind,' and go back to getting turned on again."

"Won't I just lose it again?"

"Maybe, maybe not."

"You really think it's just my negativity that's making me turn off?"

"That's my guess. The sexual mind can't tolerate much criticism."

"Why not?" she asks.

"Because it's a two-year-old."

She rolls her eyes again, and gives me a doubtful look. But I'm a lot less worried. I finally feel like I know what's going on.

The Immediate and the Remote

You'll remember in Chapter 2 we mentioned Avodah Offit, the New York psychiatrist and sex therapist who first wrote seriously about the sexual self in the 1970s. As we discussed, Offit was one of two famous sex therapists on the Upper East Side of Manhattan in those days.

Her more famous colleague, Helen Kaplan, had a more enduring influence on the field. Masters and Johnson had invented the field of sex therapy a decade earlier. Couples from all over the world would fly to Masters and Johnson's clinic in St. Louis, where they would be seen intensively for two weeks. Kaplan's 1974 book *The New Sex Therapy* showed therapists how Masters and Johnson's ideas could be adapted by local practitioners in their offices. No need to fly to St. Louis anymore to get help.

Like Masters and Johnson, Kaplan insisted that most sexual problems could be treated relatively quickly in the office. That was a revolutionary idea. But the *most* radical notion was that sexual symptoms could be treated *at all*.

At the time, most mental health specialists thought sex problems were so deeply rooted that it would be foolish to try to treat them directly. For decades, therapists had been trying to resolve people's sex symptoms by helping them resolve childhood concerns—such as Jill's confusing relationship with her mother. Following Kaplan, we sex therapists call these kinds of things "remote causes."

The radical idea that Kaplan got from Masters and Johnson was that the remote causes don't matter as much as what you're doing in the here and now that perpetuates the problem—what Kaplan called the "immediate causes."

If you can properly identify the immediate causes of someone's sexual problems, you sometimes don't have to spend years revisiting their childhoods. You can help them right away.

In order to do that, though, you need a very precise view of exactly what's going on in bed. That's where most therapists fail their clients when it comes to sex. They don't work hard enough to find the immediate causes.

The *immediate* cause of Jill's problem is this:

When she loses sexual arousal during intercourse, she responds by doing a really unnatural thing—*forcing herself to have an orgasm under circumstances where she's really more upset than turned on*. If you've been paying attention the last few chapters, you know that's not going to end well.

What Jill needs is a kinder and gentler way to react when she loses arousal.

As sex therapists, we're always looking to make sex easier. You'll usually get better results with kindness and understanding than with force.

Sex therapy, as I'm always telling my patients, is the art of the easy. You're not looking to build character. You just want to have a good time.

One Week Later

The next time Jill comes to my office she has a big smile.

"It worked," she announces.

"That's great," I say. "Tell me everything."

"I tried being gentle with myself like you said. I kept telling myself there's nothing wrong with me. That really helped me relax and just enjoy the moment. It felt like such a relief."

"Were you able to stay excited?"

"No, I lost it—as usual. But I decided not to worry about it, and I just let him come. Then I gave myself an orgasm afterward by grinding on him. He didn't seem to mind. It was just so nice to feel okay about myself during sex. It was wonderful."

"Good for you," I tell her. "Did you use your fantasy?"

"Actually, yes. But I thought about what you said, that it probably got started a long time ago when I was young and scared, and that it probably helped me feel less alone. I decided that's not such a bad thing."

"No, not at all."

"I really want to thank you for helping me see that."

"Hey, that's what I'm here for."

She smiles and rolls her eyes at me one more time. I'm going to miss that.

ANTs

There's an old joke that goes something like this:

Someone is standing in line at a pharmacy with a box of condoms and some aspirin.

The person behind them taps them on the shoulder and says, "Excuse me, but why do you do it if it makes you sick?"

Many people worry obsessively about themselves during love-making, then wonder why they're not enjoying sex. Negative obsessions about ourselves must serve some general purpose. Maybe to keep us on our guard so we don't get too carried away and do stupid things. But in bed they can cause all sorts of trouble.

Some therapists refer to negative obsessions about yourself as "Automatic Negative Thoughts." That's a term I like, mostly because of its colorful acronym—ANTs. ANTs can ruin a sexual experience just like real ants can spoil a picnic.

ANTs are perfectly designed to get your attention. If you write them down on paper, they usually look like headlines from a tabloid.

"Hopeless."

"Loser."

Hey, that's what gets them on the front page.

And they're all about *you*. What could be more interesting?

Many sex books offer techniques on how to deal with ANTs in bed. But most of these just consist of positive affirmations—replacing bad thoughts with good ones. Many of these books come from the West Coast, so I assume this kind of thing works in California. But affirmations don't cut it in New York.

Here in Manhattan the only thing that seems to work is just to realize it's an ANT and get over it.

The more attention you lavish on ANTs, the more your mind thinks they must be important. They become like celebrities—famous for being famous.

The trick, as you may have guessed, is not to give your ANTs so much emotional attention. You want them to become like former celebrities that nobody cares about anymore.

Now when Jill starts to lose arousal, she just tells Peter, "Oh it's nothing. I'm just obsessing. Hold me a minute, until it goes away." And it usually does.

Jill still comes to see me now and then. In case you're wondering, yes, she still does go back sometimes to visit the wicked man. He's always more than happy to lock her up. But now it's something she can play with and enjoy.

Hey, not everyone has the ability to get kinky like that. It can be a kind of gift—once you stop hating it so much.

It's still painful for Jill to remember all the time she spent waiting for her mother to come home. At such times, she's grateful to have Peter to hold on to. Sometimes the feeling makes her want to have sex with him. There's something reassuring about being held when she's sad.

I'm glad that when Jill first came to see me I knew enough to start with "immediate causes." When your sexual self is at its most discouraged, you need to see results quickly. That gives you hope. There'll be time later to talk about troublesome memories, since those will usually be with you for life.

There's an old cartoon about therapy. A man walks into a therapist's office with a monkey on his head. A few frames later, he walks out with the monkey on a leash.

Working with remote causes from your childhood can be like that. You never actually get rid of the monkey. But it's good to get it off your head.

Vacation Sex

It's no accident that many couples have their best sex on vacation. Vacation sex is closer to the sex we were designed for.

Humans weren't built to work long hours. It's unclear whether our early ancestors would have understood the idea of "work" at all. Your sexual self still has no idea what the word means.

Sex is essentially a leisure activity. But for most of the Manhattan couples I see, especially those raising children, the idea of leisure is just a quaint memory. As one patient of mine, a married attorney with three kids, puts it, "My weekday consists of thirteen hours of work, seven hours of sleep, and four hours left over for everything else—bathing, eating, transportation, and administration. There's not much time for conversation, much less sex."

Most busy working couples need to establish regular times for sex. Otherwise it just won't happen.

But eros can't be just put on a schedule and told to show up. If you want to stay erotically connected, you also have to cultivate erotic feeling at other times.

Fortunately there's an easy way to do this, even when you're tired.

Don't worry. It won't take much time at all.

All you need is to learn to simmer.

Getting Practical:
Sexual Arousal for Its Own Sake

A man is about to leave the house in the morning to go to work. Kissing his wife goodbye, he buries his face in her hair to inhale her scent. His arms circle her waist to pull her closer. Her body molds to his, and they breathe together for a moment, both feeling excited. Then he looks at his watch and hurries off, waving goodbye to her.

What is this couple doing?

In sex therapy we call it "simmering." Simmering means taking a quick moment to feel excited with your partner, even under conditions where sex is not going to be practical. That generally means no orgasms, no rhythmic stroking, no heavy breathing. Nothing that's going to leave you too frustrated after you have to stop.

Couples who are overworked and distracted (i.e., most of us) often neglect to get aroused in each other's company unless they intend to have sex. That's a mistake.

Most couples need to get aroused together much more frequently than that. In sex therapy we often counsel people to enjoy brief moments of arousal together for no reason at all, except that it feels good.

Teenagers simmer all the time. Here's a classic example:

Two young people are high school sweethearts. During a five-minute break between classes, they meet at a prearranged spot. They smile, kiss, stroke each other's hair, and enjoy each other's scent. They embrace and their bodies mold together. Then the bell rings. They hold each other's gaze for a long moment, steal one more kiss, then run off in different directions.

You remember the feeling, right? You get to your next class feeling somewhat buzzed. The intoxication, of course, is sexual arousal in action—making you just a little more distracted than usual.

There's no reason that older couples can't get just as distracted in the privacy of their own bedrooms and kitchens. All that's necessary is to recognize that there's more to sexual arousal than just sex.

Simmering helps cultivate the right kind of *erotic climate* in a relationship. Most couples' erotic climate is sustained more by simmering than by sex.

At the end of the day, two minutes getting excited together before falling asleep can do a lot to keep your sexual self happy. Grind up against your partner in bed and say, "This is just simmering, okay?"

Chances are, they'll be happy for the attention.

A Crucial Difference

Don't confuse simmering with "cuddling." Simmering is good for your sex life together. Cuddling not so much.

Too many couples spend their evenings curled together in front of the TV, quietly depleting whatever erotic charge might remain between them.

Too much cuddling can neuter your relationship. I'd rather couples not touch each other so much, unless there's some erotic energy to be passed around.

Some people cuddle rather than simmer, because they're afraid of frustrating their partners. They forget that physical intimacy *should* be a little frustrating. That's what keeps you in the game. It's okay. You don't have to return your partner to a state of quiescence every time they get excited.

Some wives try not to do anything that would give their husbands an erection. They assume that if they were responsible for him getting hard, then they're obligated to give him an orgasm.

That's ridiculous. We men *like* being hard. It's not a painful condition.

Erections come and go. Not every erection has to end in orgasm. If your man doesn't know this, he needs to learn it.

~~~

Instead of kissing your partner goodbye in the morning, why not simmer them goodbye? Hold them close for a bit longer than usual. Inhale the scent of their hair. There's a moment here that won't come again.

Yes, I know you're anxious about the day ahead.

But this is important too.

One or two minutes to simmer, on the way out the door in the morning. A pretty good recipe for keeping an erotic connection, for even the most harried modern couple.

The payoff in good lovemaking later can be dramatic.

Just heat and serve.

6

Two Roads to Orgasm

Great lovemaking leads to great orgasms.
Not the other way around.

*" . . . and then I asked him with my eyes to ask again yes
and then he asked me would I yes to say yes and first I put my
arms around him yes and drew him down to me so he could feel
my breasts all perfume yes and his heart was going like mad
and yes I said yes I will Yes."*
—JAMES JOYCE, *ULYSSES*

What's for Dessert?

We sex therapists aren't so interested in orgasms. We're among
the few humans on the planet who aren't. One of my favorite defi-
nitions of a sex therapist is someone who spends most of their professional life urging couples not to make too big a fuss about
orgasms.

Why not? Because in really good sex, orgasm should be like dessert at the end of a good meal. Memorable, perhaps. But not the
reason you went out to dinner.

In my experience, the couples that have the best sex are the ones
who *don't* set orgasm as a goal. They just enjoy it—if and when it
comes.

Now you might think I'm crazy to minimize the importance of orgasms. Especially when nearly every other sex book in the world is promising you bigger and better ones.

But eros, as I've mentioned, doesn't like goals. It's usually an advantage if you can focus on *turn-ons* instead.

Then, if you're lucky, after you've eaten and enjoyed everything on your plate, suddenly the dessert tray appears and you realize, "OMG, I forgot! There's gonna be DESSERT!"

You've had that happen a few times, right?

Dessert just kind of finishes you off. That's how an orgasm should be.

You can't survive on just dessert. A lot of couples try to satisfy each other with orgasms, then they wonder why they're still hungry.

But I LIKE Dessert!

Yes, I know you do. And there are times when a good orgasm can be just the thing if you're restless or need help getting to sleep. But you didn't need to read this book to figure that out! Aren't we after a bigger prize here?

In really good lovemaking, orgasm is just punctuation at the end of the sentence. After orgasm, most men lose all interest in sex. For women, the punctuation of orgasm tends to be less emphatic—a comma maybe, instead of a period. After orgasm most women still remain capable of sexual feeling. For most men, it's pretty much zero.

For this reason, a woman should generally be first to have dessert. As a sex therapist I've heard too many stories where the man has his orgasm first and then spends a long time trying to bring his wife to climax. This leads to all sorts of mischief.

She knows he's just waiting for her to finish so he can go to sleep or turn the TV back on. Which of course isn't much of an aphrodisiac for her.

The quest to give your partner an orgasm is the chief cause of a lot of bad sex. You wouldn't sit down to eat just in order to have dessert, would you?

Okay, maybe *sometimes* you would. But you wouldn't want to make a habit of it, right?

Best not to make a habit of it in bed either.

Two Roads to Orgasm

Whether an orgasm turns out to be really worthwhile depends on the intensity of the arousal that preceded it. Great arousal leads naturally to great orgasms. But most of us are also perfectly capable of having orgasms without much arousal at all.

One might say there's a high road and a low road to orgasm. Approached from the high road, orgasm is just an afterthought, like dessert at the end of a memorable meal.

The low road is where you're not very aroused, but the right kind of friction in the right spot can still make you come. But those orgasms don't count for much and can leave you chronically hungry.

Sometimes an orgasm can be a sort of giving up. As in, "Well, I'm not going to get much more excited than I am right now, so let's get this over with." Low-road orgasms can be useful once in a while for relieving anxiety, putting you to sleep, or momentarily quelling unwanted sexual thoughts. But I encourage you not to take the low road too often. Better just to skip dessert, if you can.

If it feels like you're *not even close* to orgasm, don't push it.

If it feels like work, don't do it.

Sex should never feel like work, as you know.

If you're not really feeling excited during sex with your partner, don't just expect them to have to get you off. That's not fair to either of you.

Okay, if you simply *have* to have dessert so you won't be all cranky later, then why not just give yourself an orgasm in bed with your partner? That can be plenty erotic if you do it right—as we'll see at the end of Chapter 9.

But don't make a big thing about it.

Remember, it's just dessert.

Boy-gasms and Girl-gasms

Lately I've spoken to several women who disagree passionately with me about orgasm. They tell me it's definitely *not* dessert. They say their orgasms *totally* qualify as a main course.

I've begun to wonder whether these women's orgasms might represent something truly different that we men aren't privy to.

Male-to-female transgender activist and writer Julia Serano writes that when she first started taking female hormones, her experience of physical intimacy was like nothing she'd ever felt as a man. On estrogen, when she kissed or nuzzled her wife, "it felt as though fireworks were going off in my brain."

Her experience of climax changed as well. She writes, "I found that I could go way beyond what used to be the point of orgasm, writhing for fifteen minutes in a sexual state that was far more intense than I had ever experienced before."

Serano is careful to note that others' experiences might be different, but she says her current "girl-gasms"—as she calls them—are way more intense than her "boy-gasms" ever were. "Each one has a different flavor and intensity," she reports. "They are less centralized and more diffuse throughout my body, and they are often multiple."

Many women say they can get "boy-gasms" too, if they just want something quick. But very few men seem to be able to achieve the kind of "girl-gasms" that Serano describes.

In Greek mythology, a man named Tiresias was said to have lived part of his life as a woman. People were always pumping Tiresias for information about who enjoyed sex more—men or women.

Tiresias would always tell everybody that his best-gasms had been his girl-gasms.

Getting to Yes

In a word, the female orgasm is "yes." It's a big, gloriously large, wet, wonderful, resounding "yes." . . . At least once in her sex life, a woman should experience the full and frank pleasure of releasing the word "yes" as loudly and for as long as her lungs will allow.

—KATHERINE FEENEY, "SAYING YES TO THE FEMALE ORGASM"

Among women of a certain tribal village, the term most commonly used to describe an orgasm apparently translates to something like, "*Yes! Yes!*"

It's the same thing in the developed West. Something about that little word "yes" seems to connect to female orgasm in a deep way.

Maybe it's because women have to learn very early to say "no." Don't make unnecessary eye contact. Cross your legs. Don't say "yes" on the first date.

As a rule, men don't have that "no" thing going on so much. But for a woman to say "yes" in a wholehearted way is a big deal.

Of course it's not always so easy to get to "yes." Male and female alike, we all have sexual accelerators and sexual brakes. But most women tend to have more sensitive brakes. Their erotic minds are naturally more inclined to say "no" unless certain conditions are met. This seems to be true for all aspects of most women's sexual response—from orgasm to arousal to desire.

Some women feel uncomfortable really letting go enough to climax. For example, it's not uncommon for a mother of small children to be worried she'll be too distracted if one of her kids needs her. Sometimes very competent childcare will do the trick. More often a trip to a bed-and-breakfast is called for.

Emily Nagoski, author of the recent bestselling sex book *Come as You Are*, likens all the various parts of a woman's mind to a flock of birds. To get to a really wholehearted "yes," you have to get enough birds flying in the same direction.

There's also the practice factor. Most women need some experience masturbating to get really good at having orgasms. If so, you actually couldn't have picked a better time to learn. There are now fabulous resources available online (see Notes).

Science has also now cleared up some misunderstandings about female orgasm that have befuddled people for centuries. We now know, for example, that the clitoris—not the vagina—is where a woman's orgasms typically "happen." But most of the clitoris is internal, so it's easy to get confused.

The clitoris you can see at the top of a woman's vulva is simply the command center for her "inner clitoris," a vast underground arousal system that reaches out to her entire vulva, her vagina, and beyond. So-called vaginal orgasms really just come from stimulating the inner clitoris indirectly through intercourse.

The fact that a woman has both an outer clitoris and an inner one means you can stimulate them both at the same time. Sometimes that can be just the ticket.

Even with superb technique, though, many women still can't reliably reach orgasm. Some women just decide to enjoy sex knowing they're not going to get dessert. But vibrators and other sex toys just keep getting better and better. These days more and more women (and an increasing number of men) use them to make orgasm easier.

Is this a good thing? I think so. But I happen to be biased in favor of easy—as you know. If you need a vibrator to make getting to orgasm less of an ordeal, I say go for it.

Just remember to bring the appropriate adaptors if you travel internationally.

The Two-Step

Remember Carmen and Scott from Chapter 2? As you'll recall, their big problem was that Scott kept trying to give Carmen an orgasm, but her sexual self wasn't cooperating. Her sexual self was too busy worrying about whether she'd damaged herself by masturbating so much with the running water in the bathtub.

Once Carmen realized that she wasn't in fact damaged, she began to enjoy giving herself orgasms in bed with Scott. Once in a while she managed it during intercourse too—though that was more hit-or-miss.

Carmen didn't really care. She liked that sex with Scott made her feel good about herself. Which to me is a pretty nice definition of good sex.

Carmen and Scott stayed married, bought an apartment in Brooklyn, and went on to have three children. Several years later Carmen came to see me again with her youngest child asleep in a stroller. She got out her phone and showed me pictures of her growing family, and we chatted for a while about nannies and pediatricians and what-not. Then we got down to talking about sex.

She said she wasn't sure whether or not she and Scott were still on good footing there. They still had sex, but it was only once a week—early on Sunday mornings before the children woke up.

"Do you think that's enough?" she asked, clearly worried.

"Does it feel like enough for you?" I asked her.

"To tell you the truth," she said, "I'd be totally fine if we skipped it and I just got another half hour of sleep. But sex is important to Scott, so I guess it's important for me too."

"When you have sex, do you get excited?" I asked.

"Not as much as before we had kids, when my body was younger and I wasn't tired all the time. But yeah, I can get into it."

"How about orgasms?"

"Not even close. Scott always has one, but he's learned not to pressure me about it."

"Do you still masturbate?" I asked.

"Sometimes Scott will take the kids out for the afternoon, and I'll do some yoga at home and then masturbate afterward."

I asked her whether the yoga helped, and she said she thought it helped her get back into her body. She said that when she focused on her breath, she would sometimes feel a stillness inside—pleasant and welcome, like something reflected on the still surface of a lake.

Most of the time, she realized, her mind was too agitated to experience that stillness—as if someone were splashing around in the water. But if she kept bringing her focus gently back to her breathing, the choppy water would eventually calm enough for it to return.

The stillness she described wasn't exactly horniness. But it opened her to pleasure—and then one thing usually led to another.

"Did you ever consider doing that breathing thing before you have sex with Scott?" I ask her.

"No. Do you think it would help?"

I told her I thought it might help quiet her mind. She liked the idea but she said she wasn't sure what that would look like, exactly, in bed with Scott.

"Just lie next to him and focus on your breathing," I told her. "Let everything get as still as possible. Feel the weight of your body on the mattress. Inhale the scent of your bodies in bed. That's step one."

"Is that supposed to get me aroused?"

"No. It's just supposed to get you focused."

"Okay, I like it so far. Tell me about step two."

"Step two is to hold on to that stillness and let it be the foundation for your arousal. Tell Scott not to touch you. Just have him lie quietly while you touch *him*. This is just for you. It's selfish."

"I think he's going to like this a lot. Is it okay if it leads to sex?"

"Sure, but remember—if it does, it's still part of step two. Hold on to that quiet feeling inside."

"Are there any more steps?"

"No. Only two. First tune in to the silence of your own body, then stay in that silence when you make love."

"Okay," she said. "I'm intrigued."

The results were spectacular. Carmen enjoyed step one so much that she almost didn't want to proceed to step two. Sometimes when Scott was tired, she just enjoyed the stillness of step one for its own sake.

But when they were both rested, by the time she started on step two her sexual self would often be feeling so quiet and happy that when Scott got excited and wanted to make love she was fully open to it.

The whole thing was definitely sexier. Often it lasted all the way to orgasm. And the orgasms were typically much more satisfying.

"Does this thing have a name?" Carmen asked a few weeks later in my office.

"Let's just call it the 'Two-Step.'"

"Did you discover it?"

"People are always discovering it. You discovered it yourself by noticing how yoga got you in the mood for an orgasm. I just suggested you do the same thing in bed with Scott."

It's normal for a couple to lose their erotic inspiration and to have to look for it again, as we'll see in Chapters 15 and 16. It's absolutely crucial when you go looking for it that you first look within yourself.

If Carmen had consulted most of the sex books on the shelf at Barnes & Noble, she'd have probably been told to try fantasy, or leather, or porn. And in fairness those things can sometimes gain you a few weeks of excitement.

But they usually fade quickly, because they don't address the fundamental problem of the sexual self trying to find its way home.

The Inner Game of Sex

When the mind is free of any thought or judgment, it is still and acts like a mirror. Then and only then can we know things as they are.
—W. TIMOTHY GALLWEY, THE INNER GAME OF TENNIS

One of Masters and Johnson's key contributions was that arousal either happens or it doesn't, based on the conditions of the moment. You can't control it. The best you can do is to get out of its way.

That's true of a lot of other things too. In 1983, tennis pro W. Timothy Gallwey wrote *The Inner Game of Tennis* to help people learn to play better tennis by getting out of their own way and letting their natural instincts take over. The book went on to sell over a million copies—so Gallwey was clearly on to something bigger than tennis. It's still in print, and I recommend it to my sex therapy patients all the time.

Years ago when I first started teaching the Two-Step to couples, I had no idea I was part of a broad movement that included *The Inner Game* and that would eventually sweep through the mental health field like a brushfire on dry grass—the "*mindfulness*" movement.

Mindfulness is based on traditional Buddhist meditation. But it isn't as esoteric as you might think. It doesn't require you to sit cross-legged, or eat vegan, or do anything you wouldn't do normally.

Mindfulness is just something that happens naturally when you *pay attention to the present moment, without judgment.* That's a skill that requires practice—whether you're getting ready to play tennis or to have sex. You can't learn it from a book.

The word "mindfulness" doesn't sound at first like something you'd associate with sex. ("*Mindlessness*" might seem a better choice.) But if you look again carefully at the definition of mindfulness two paragraphs above, you'll see three things that we know are essential for good sex:

Like mindfulness, sex is all about *paying attention.*

It's all about the *present moment.*

And it's all about *being without judgment* (that is, acceptance).

The opposite of mindfulness isn't mindlessness. On the contrary, it's *getting too attached to your own thoughts.*

If you don't get too attached to your thoughts, then your mind naturally switches over to a state of simple mindful awareness. That's what Carmen managed to do with her quiet breathing, and it can be a powerful facilitator of arousal. That state of mindful awareness is where all the good stuff happens.

Anything at all can be a mindfulness practice, as long as it helps you to be in the moment. Many women have been doing mindfulness for years as a part of preparing for sex, without having a name for it. Getting undressed, taking a bath, putting on a favorite fragrance, these can all be wonderful mindfulness practices if you do them right.

Dr. Lori Brotto, who's the Canada research chair in Women's Sexual Health at the University of British Columbia in Vancouver, came up with the idea of applying mindfulness to sex in 2003, and together with her research team she's been testing and refining it ever since.

Her eight-week Mindfulness-Based Sex Therapy (MBST) groups always start in the same way: with everyone eating a raisin. Actually, you only eat it after first spending some time giving the raisin your whole focus—something most of us don't ordinarily do.

Women often report never having had such a good time eating a raisin before, and that it was nice to pay attention to just one thing for a change. They then apply this kind of focused attention to their breath, as Carmen did. Then to their bodies, to sounds, and eventually to their thoughts and their vulvas.

Vulvar mindfulness is not exactly masturbation, since it has no goal in mind. But with practice, it can lead to all sorts of good things.

Mindfulness naturally leads you in a mystical direction. But didn't we always kind of know that about sex as well? As Emily Nagoski writes toward the end of *Come as You Are*, "It's about what happens when you make contact with the peace at the center and core of yourself, which is the same peace at the center and core of the universe."

Whether you get deeply involved with mindfulness or just limit yourself to a quick Two-Step in bed with your partner, it's worth knowing that in each moment there are riches waiting to be discovered. The world is full of small wonders, and sex can be one of them if you allow it.

As I mentioned, we sex therapists aren't that interested in orgasms. But we're very interested in what road you take to get there.

Some roads are infinitely better than others.

PART II

Women and Men

Female or male, we all want to be accepted, enjoyed, and told we are wonderful. But beyond this fundamental level, male and female sexual selves tend to differ.

In Part II, we're going to discuss some of these differences—and the mischief they often cause when women and men become partners. We'll also talk about same-sex relationships. But our main focus will be on male-female couples, since they're the most common and in many ways the most troublesome.

Be forewarned, though. Gender is a hard subject. Anatomical gender tends to be straightforward, but masculinity and femininity are culturally defined and extremely complex.

There are exceptions to every generalization you could make about gender. Female and male are neither opposites nor mutually exclusive. Look closely enough and most of us turn out to be "gender-benders" in one way or another.

Writing about gender is a formidable and risky task. Because of this, most sex books either focus exclusively on one gender, or else they try to be unisex.

But a great many problems of erotic life arise from the ordinary erotic differences between men and women. These problems make up a large part of every sex therapist's practice.

This being so, there comes a point as a sex writer where you have to either face the issue head-on, or forever regret your lack of courage.

We've come to that point now.
Shall we proceed?
All those in favor, turn the page.

The Woman in the Mirror

Most women have a fundamental need to feel desired.
So do most men, of course.
But for most women it's more of a "thing."

"It is better to be looked over, than overlooked."
—MAE WEST

One day at a swimming pool in Miami with my kids, I notice a small group of eleven-year-old girls run over to where an eleven-year-old boy is swimming with his father. One of the girls points to one of her friends and asks the boy, "My friend Kathy wants to know if you think she's sexy."

The girls run off, giggling. The boy rolls his eyes, but keeps an eye on the girls.

Moments later, Kathy returns to the pool wearing a bright yellow bikini bathing suit. The girls come prancing back to the boy, showing off the bikini bathing suit with Kathy inside it.

The boy pretends to be bothered by all this attention, but proceeds to execute several beautiful flip turns. He demonstrates all of the swimming strokes he knows, and then makes a big splash in the water—getting all the girls just a little bit wet. They run off giggling again. Everyone seems to be having a very good time.

These children are too young to do much more than go through the preliminary motions, but you can already see the form that courtship will take later on.

Her focus is broader. She's interested in his response, of course. But she's also quite fascinated by her own body, and by her own bikini.

She tries to get his attention by showing what she *has*—or more precisely, who she *is*. His behavior emphasizes instead what he's capable of *doing*. In the conventional form of the heterosexual mating dance, *being* is a quintessentially female activity, and *doing* is a quintessentially male one.

It's amazing how often the media get this wrong. Men's magazines, for example, tend to feature endless articles on how to get a perfectly sculpted body. This is for the most part a waste of time.

Sure, six-pack abs look impressive. But they'll hold most women's attention for a few minutes at most. A man with great abs who can't hold a conversation (or a job) isn't going to interest many women for very long.

And women's magazines go on and on about "killer moves" that will light a man's fire in bed. Equally a waste of time.

Whether or not a woman has "killer moves" in bed is largely irrelevant to most men unless she fundamentally turns him on. The eleven-year-old girl's question at the pool hits the nail right on the head: "Do you think I'm sexy?"

What a woman *does* with her sexiness doesn't matter as much.

The other thing we should notice is that the boy's actions are somewhat aggressive. He instinctively knows it's okay to splash his admirers a bit, and they love him for it. It's been a bit boring for them, strutting around the pool all day. Some raw male energy helps make the afternoon more interesting.

In adult male-female relationships this male energy is often the first thing to disappear. In the next several chapters we'll talk about why—and what can be done about it.

Many straight women in my office tell me they go half crazy waiting day after day for their male partners to show them any real passion. A man is more likely than a woman to be dragged to sex therapy by an exasperated partner who complains that he no longer seems to be "present."

Not much has been written about this problem. Sex advice for women has traditionally focused on things you can control: how to stop criticizing your body, how to heal from past trauma, how to speak up about your sexual needs, how to reach climax more often, how to have sex so it doesn't hurt.

Women tend to be good at taking responsibility for relationships. Sometimes too much so. The one thing a woman can't control— the quality of her partner's attention to her—hasn't received nearly enough consideration.

The Conventional Script

Sex in male-female couples tends to follow a conventional script that's been around for a long time. It's the same script that governs traditional couples' dancing. You know, the kind you see couples do competitively on TV.

He leads, and she follows. He is in charge, but she's the main object of attention.

Sex is traditionally organized along similar lines. He's expected to initiate and take charge. If he refuses, it can be a problem—like having a male dance partner who won't lead.

He tends to worry about his performance. Her body is the main attraction, and accordingly her biggest concern is usually her appearance.

The conventional script doesn't have much to say about gay or lesbian mating. Gays and lesbians have historically had the advantage of being able to write their own rules.

But pieces of this script seem to be wired into the erotic brains of most straight people. Despite all the changes in men's and women's lives over the past few decades, heterosexual couples still tend to follow it rather closely.

There are signs that the script might be shifting a bit these days. Women seem to have become more avid connoisseurs of *men's* bodies. And more women now actively pursue sex for its own sake.

But to me these seem like novelties. I'm not convinced much has really changed. Straight women in my office still prefer men who are confident and decisive. In bed, they still expect them to make the first move. And they still spend much more time worrying about how they look.

I think it's possible that a hundred years from now, in parts of the developed West, we'll have produced a society where gender roles are much less predictable. In such a society, those dance competitions on TV will probably look odd.

But I'm not holding my breath waiting for that to happen. I believe sex for most heterosexual couples will continue to look more or less like traditional couples' dancing for some time to come.

You might consider the chapters that follow to be a series of dance lessons. They won't necessarily get you a prize on TV. But they might keep you from stepping on each other's toes.

The Woman in the Mirror

An elderly woman comes to see me about some problems with her husband. At some point in our conversation she mentions that in the early years of their marriage the sex they shared was particularly good.

"What was so good about it?" I ask, naturally curious.

She answers without a moment's hesitation.

"I felt pretty," she says. "And I felt sexy."

A lot has changed of course since this woman was a newlywed. It's now recognized that there's much more to a woman's sexual pleasure than simply being the object of desire.

But many women in my office still tell me that feeling desired is more important than orgasm. They still read magazines with names like *Glamour* and *Allure*. And they still enjoy fantasies of being sexually irresistible.

We men don't focus on our physical attractiveness the same way—at least not publicly. But a woman can buy a magazine called *Self* and no one thinks that's weird.

I don't know how much of this is biological and how much cultural. It's certain that culture amplifies gender differences. (Those kids at the pool are no doubt acting out what they've seen on TV.) But women's preoccupation with their physical bodies is so powerful that I think some of it must be inborn.

Are women more erotically narcissistic? No. Anyone who's ever treated a man for an erection problem knows that men can be extremely narcissistic in bed too. But there's something particularly self-reflective about female eroticism, and I don't think we've figured it out yet.

Look at the newsstands:

Who's on the covers of men's magazines? Mostly beautiful women.

How about the covers of *women's* magazines?

Hmm. *Beautiful women.*

What's this all about?

A Room Full of Women

It's spring in Chicago, and I'm standing in a big meeting room surrounded by women. I'm having a wonderful time—especially because we're all talking about sex.

It's the annual spring meeting of the Society for Sex Therapy and Research (SSTAR)—one of the world's preeminent sex organizations. The gender ratio at sex therapy meetings tends to be fairly lopsided in favor of women. This one is no exception. For some reason, women just seem to be more interested in sex. Or at least in thinking about it.

I'm especially interested this year to hear my colleague Dr. Marta Meana from the University of Nevada, Las Vegas present her new research on something she calls "Erotic Self-Focus."

It's long been known that women get easily turned off by *negative* feelings about their bodies. But how about the opposite: Might a woman's *positive* feelings about her body be a big contributor to her arousal?

Meana and her graduate student Evan Fertel conducted a study where they asked male and female subjects questions like,

> *"Is it arousing for you to imagine stripping in front of many members of the opposite sex?"*
> *"Does the very thought of being a man or a woman turn you on?"*
> *"Does looking at yourself in the mirror in your undergarments help get you in the mood for sex?"*
> *"Would you want to have sex with yourself?"*

The results were clear. Many more women than men said "yes" to these questions.

Men often seemed not to know what to do with questions like, "Would you want to have sex with yourself?" But a lot of women understood the question immediately, and replied that they'd very much like to.

Meana is a careful scientist. When I talk with her in Chicago, she keeps emphasizing that her results are preliminary—and that future studies will be needed to refine these concepts. But I think this line of research points to something people have known intuitively for a long time.

It also explains why women's magazines feature pictures of beautiful women. The pictures on the page are intended to stimulate your enjoyment of what you see in your own mirror.

Yes, I know they're also intended to make you buy lots of beauty products. But the beauty industry didn't get this big for nothing.

Pop vocalist Katy Perry had a hit song, "Teenage Dream," a few years back, where she sang,

Let you put your hands on me
In my skintight jeans
Be your teenage dream tonight.

Now if this were a young man, he'd more likely be singing about his *partner's* jeans, not his own. There are hundreds of country songs that praise women for looking good in denim.

But for the young woman in the Katy Perry song, her boyfriend's greatest value is that she's *his* teenage dream—and that he likes to put his hands on her when she's wearing those jeans of hers.

You don't have to be a sex therapist to know that a woman's sexual enjoyment strongly depends on how she thinks she looks in her jeans.

Melissa

A few weeks ago Melissa stood at the mirror, looked herself up and down, and puzzled over the changes in her marriage in the three years since their wedding. Her body seemed pretty much the same, as far as she could tell. But her husband, Rob, no longer took the same kind of interest in it.

They still had sex once a week or so, but something was definitely missing.

After her session in the mirror, Melissa decided she didn't want to live like this anymore. But when she mentioned the idea of seeing someone about their sex life, Rob's answer was an emphatic no. After some tense arguments about this, she decided to come in by herself.

"When we were first married, he couldn't keep his hands off me," she says, trying not to cry. "Now it's like he couldn't care less."

What might be going on? We both wonder.

Maybe he's just not attracted to her anymore. Maybe he's suffering from depression, or low testosterone. Or perhaps it's an extramarital affair, a pituitary tumor, or some complicated emotional thing from his childhood. The possibilities are endless.

"The patient is the couple," we're all told in training. But what to do when only half a couple shows up in the office?

All therapists know this situation well. The person who's in distress comes for help, while the person *causing* the distress is content to stay at home.

There *is* a solution to this problem, but it involves a bit of bluffing.

Tricks of the Trade

"Here's what you might do," I say to Melissa. "Tell him you plan to see me by yourself, every week—and that Dr. Snyder says this might take *years*."

"You're kidding, right?" she asks.

"Half kidding," I say. "But that'll get his attention."

"Then what?"

"Tell him if he wants it to go faster, he needs to show up."

She giggles.

"You're right. That *is* a bit of a bluff."

"Sure. But it also happens to be true."

She says she'll think about it. And I make sure to allocate some extra time for her next appointment, just in case he decides to come in with her.

One Week Later

The next week Melissa and Rob arrive together. He's a nice-looking businessman in a well-fitting suit. He looks me over, warily.

"I don't understand why she's so upset," he says. "We have sex, and it's usually good. What's the problem?"

Melissa turns to him, exasperated. "The problem is that it's always me initiating."

"What's wrong with that?" he asks. "You know I'm always willing."
She looks flummoxed.

"I want you to *want* me."

"I do," he insists.

"I don't feel it," she says.

It seems strange that Rob doesn't understand what Melissa is saying. Is he just playing dumb? *Almost all* straight women want their partners to take the initiative. Doesn't everybody know this?

Sure, a woman may initiate sex once in a while, just for fun. But it's important for most women to know they never *have* to initiate unless they want to.

Maybe Rob just doesn't understand this yet. It seems unbelievable that the problem could just be ignorance on his part. But hey, let's start simple and see where it takes us.

"You know, Rob," I say, "what Melissa is saying is pretty much what I hear from most women. They like sex, but the thing they really crave is to feel desired."

He weighs my words.

"That doesn't seem right to me," he says. "We have a pretty equitable relationship. Why should it always be on me to initiate?"

"I agree it's not exactly fair," I say. "But that's just how things are. Sex is like a game of tennis. You're the man. It's pretty much always your serve."

"Still doesn't seem fair."

"I told you—it's not."

He's not buying this. Feeling stuck, I decide to try another approach.

Rat Sex

"Look," I say. "Let me tell you how rats do it."

"Rats?"

"Yeah. Just stay with me on this one. We sex therapists happen to be very interested in how rats do it. Especially the foreplay."

Rob and Melissa look at me with curiosity, waiting to hear about rat foreplay.

This had better be good.

"Here's what happens," I tell them. "The female rat goes in front of the male rat and flashes her rear end in front of him. If all goes well, he runs after her. He has to chase her around and around, until at some point when he's totally exhausted she decides he's chased her enough, and she finally lets him have her."

"I can see why she'd like that," says Melissa.

"Why?" asks Rob, still not quite getting it.

"Because it means he was really interested."

"Why does she care so much?"

"I don't know. We just do."

I see Rob beginning to catch on.

"So you want me . . . to *chase* you?"

"Of course!"

"That's *it*?"

"Pretty much."

"Why didn't you just *say* so?"

"I didn't have the words to say it, until he told us about the rats."

Rat Sex and Human Sex

In a recent professional book, *Treating Sexual Desire Disorders*, sex therapist and writer Esther Perel lets one of her clients, a Spanish woman, tell the story of what she calls *"Juego"*:

"You think I'm attracted to you and that you can just have me, but you're wrong. You don't have me yet . . . The more persistently you pursue me, the more attractive and irresistible I feel, which makes me move away some more to see if you'll keep coming after me, if I can make you want me even more."

This kind of thing is so foreign to the typical male mind that few men understand it at all.

Is *"Juego"* just the human version of what female rats do? We'll never be able to ask the female rats. But something about their tendency to like being chased has made more than one sex expert stand up and exclaim, "Yes, that's it!"

The problem in most marriages is that when a man starts to feel his wife is a sure thing, he stops chasing her. When that happens, their erotic relationship loses something essential.

For whatever reason, as the female partner in a heterosexual relationship you're usually the CSO (chief sexual officer): counting how many times you've made love recently, monitoring from his actions and words how strongly he desires you, and paying closer attention to the health and vitality of the sex life that the two of you share.

Sex books typically advise women to manipulate the situation—by introducing elements of risk or uncertainty, or by making themselves less reliably available. I don't particularly like that approach. Most men don't enjoy having their feelings manipulated, and most women don't appreciate being given one more job to do.

I find it's better to put the responsibility on the *man*, and to educate him about his partner's need to be pursued. Then it's his job to decide how to use this information and to face the consequences of his decisions.

Sometimes I'll tell him *he* has to become the chief sexual officer. If he can't or won't do this, then I have no pity for him. The reality is that a woman needs to feel desired. For most women, it's like oxygen.

As the chief sexual officer in the relationship, I tell him the main part of his job is to *notice* when she might be pulling away from him—and if that happens to imagine the possibility that like the female rat she might be hoping to begin a chase.

It's not always necessary to chase her all the way to the bedroom. The technique of *simmering*, which we learned about in Chapter 5, can sometimes serve just as well. When we discussed simmering earlier, it was in gender-neutral terms. But simmering is seldom a gender-neutral thing. It's far more important for you to simmer her, than for her to simmer you.

Many women very much enjoy being grabbed passionately by someone they love and desire.

But not all women do. Everyone's wiring is different, so it's usually best to ask.

It's also important to remember that women who like being grabbed usually hate being *groped*. Make sure you're really grabbing her—not groping her.

Here's how to tell the difference:

	Grabbing	Groping
Object of attention:	Whole woman	A body part
Mood:	Serious	Idle
Passion:	High	Low or nonexistent

If a partner hasn't learned the difference between grabbing and groping, then all kinds of relationship disasters can result.

A Darker Mirror

And so I started hating my body. Not just the shape of it, although there was that. I hated having a body at all. My body made it impossible for me to succeed at being a girl.
—GLENNON DOYLE, *LOVE WARRIOR*

When Marta Meana and Evan Fertel finish their presentation at SSTAR in Chicago on women's erotic self-focus, I'm interested to see what kinds of questions will be asked afterward by the mostly female audience during the question-and-answer period that follows.

For the most part the audience's questions are rather grim. Many women in the audience seem to feel there's something problematic about erotic self-focus.

As Meana sees it, a woman who enjoys erotic self-focus gains an extra ingredient for arousal. She is more independent, more self-validating. That's certainly possible, of course—especially if you have enough confidence to begin with. But the reality is that self-focus often turns negative.

Glennon Doyle Melton, in her recent memoir *Love Warrior*, writes that this happened when she was ten. "Ten is when I noticed that I was chubbier, frizzier, oilier than the other girls. I became self-conscious. My body started to feel like a separate, strange entity, and I thought it odd that people would examine and judge *me* based on what they saw, something that didn't have much to do with who I was."

From that point on, being in the world became for her an out-of-body experience, as it does for many women. No wonder there are often tears of joy and grief when much later on a woman manages to reunite with her own body.

There's also the fact that being desired can be hazardous. If a woman is lucky, her first experiences of feeling desired provide the foundation for a lifetime of validation and pleasure. But few women are so lucky.

Most women in my office have experienced some form of sexual coercion. A not insignificant number have been raped—most often by someone they knew. Almost all have at one time or another been sexually harassed. The sexualization of a woman's body can be a form of trauma, and some women repeat this trauma when they sexualize their own bodies.

"It's a cruel discovery for young girls," writes Sallie Foley in *Sex Matters for Women*, "that they are vulnerable solely because of their gender. It's equally cruel that they will have to carry into their adult years a sense of vigilance and suspicion that can interfere with their capacity to love and experience life with a sense of abandonment and joy."

Then there's figuring out how to actually enjoy sex. Women have been objects of desire for as long as people have kept records. But the conventional script has never had much to say about a woman's own sexual pleasure.

Women often tell me that sex in their teens and early twenties was mostly just for getting attention. More full-bodied pleasure in lovemaking often didn't happen until they got older—if it happened at all.

As Peggy Orenstein notes in her recent book *Girls & Sex*, young women's lives today tend to be intensely sexualized, but often at the expense of their own sexuality. The same is true for a lot of older women as well. Being pursued can be lots of fun, but there's still the question of what to do when your partner catches you. As my colleague Pamela Madsen writes, sometimes you have to drop the mirror to find out what you yourself desire.

Society both idealizes and disparages women, and sex provides a convenient vehicle for both. Men's sex lives often aren't particularly easy either—as we'll see in the chapters that follow. But women's bodies are the object of such intense scrutiny that no account of a woman's sexual psychology can be complete without considering the range of feelings she might experience when she looks in the mirror.

Men at Work

*For a man to think his partner is sexy, they don't usually
have to be doing anything in particular. But for a woman to see
a man as sexy, some action on his part is typically required.*

*"My husband and I met on a volleyball court on Fire Island.
What he remembers about that day is my teeny-weeny yellow
bikini. What I remember, besides his being tall, adorable, and a
dynamite server, is how much he made me laugh."*
—LETTY COTTIN POGREBIN, ELLE

Erotic images of women tend to feature them in a state of pleasurable relaxation—sunning by the pool, or relaxing in bed wearing
next to nothing. A smiling woman in a state of repose is a near
universal turn-on for straight men.

Male sex appeal is different. Few women want to see a hot guy
just relaxing. Most straight women like to see men *doing* things—like
fixing the dishwasher, or saving a village.

One thing that straight women universally say turns them *off* is
to see their husbands sitting around doing nothing. Which is totally unfair to us men, but that's the way it is.

Women sometimes get nervous when their husbands are facing
retirement. What's he going to *do* all day? Hang around the house?
Major turn-off.

A straight woman wants her man to be doing something valuable and important that they can both be proud of. If he makes money at it, all the better. As Avodah Offit wrote in *The Sexual Self*, "Wealth has the power to stimulate vaginal lubrication in many women who will admit to it, and in many more who will not."

Many women in my office say they dream of a man making a *grand gesture*—a noble sacrifice that proves how important she is to him. Whether it's those diamond earrings that cost three months' salary, or just something more modest like sending her flowers at work, the key thing is that he undertake some special action for her and her alone.

One common problem in relationships is that the man runs out of grand gestures and doesn't know what to do next. It's important to reassure men that simple acts of thoughtfulness can count just as much as grand gestures.

By the way, there's one "grand gesture" that as a married man you have an opportunity to do very early on. It's crucially important that you get this right. When the first conflict arises between your wife and your family of origin, she'll instinctively test you to see where your loyalties lie. If you side with her, you pass the test. If instead you give her a lecture about how she should be nicer to your family, don't be surprised if her libido suddenly drops.

A Question of Balance

In thirty years of being a sex therapist, I've rarely heard a man complain about the way a new partner kisses. But women in my office tend to talk about this a lot.

Too hard. Too soft. Too wet. Not wet enough. Too much tongue. Not enough tongue.

A kiss should be just right. Not too hard, not too soft. The elements should be in balance.

Then of course there's dental hygiene, breath quality, and whether a partner seems to be really paying attention. Most women, on kissing someone for the first time, will do a detailed assessment. There are a number of things to consider, and her level of desire may rise or fall accordingly.

When a man in my office talks to me about a new partner, it's a lot simpler. Either they turn him on, or they don't. But for most women this question can be exceedingly complex.

Few men are aware how meticulously their female partners assess their behavior. Sometimes the needle on a woman's erotic compass can swing wildly as she absorbs and considers everything about him. One discordant element can ruin the whole experience.

It's the same when she evaluates his character. He should be thoughtful, but not so thoughtful that he seems wimpy. A bit of a dominant attitude can be sexy, but not so dominant that he's pushy or domineering. A certain sophistication would be nice, but he'll need some down-to-earth values to complement it.

It can be tricky sometimes to get the balance just right.

Rat Sex, Revisited

Remember Melissa and Rob from the previous chapter? After a few weeks Rob seems to have taken my lecture on "rat sex" to heart, and has started to initiate sex with Melissa again.

But at their next appointment I find Melissa in my waiting room all alone looking very unhappy, and I know something is wrong.

"It's hopeless," she says, wiping her eyes with a tissue and trying not to smudge her makeup. "I can't go on like this."

"What happened?" I ask.

"It's Rob," she says. "I can't stand having sex with him anymore." Melissa cries some more.

"Do you think I'm bad for saying that?" she asks. "I mean, here I dragged him in to see you because he wouldn't initiate. And now he's doing everything I asked for. I'm getting wet and everything, and I'm coming all over the place. But I can't stand it."

At this moment, I have no idea what's bothering Melissa. Whatever it is, she seems to be as confused by it as I am.

An inexperienced observer might accuse Melissa of just being difficult to please. But as a sex therapist you learn to expect this kind of thing. The sexual self doesn't lie. People often don't know exactly what they want until someone tries to give it to them—and then they realize that's not it.

Let's see if we can figure out what's going on.

"Have you *always* felt this way during sex with Rob?" I ask. "Or is this something new?"

"I think it's always been there."

"What's wrong?"

"He's so *earnest* about it—like he's just trying to get a good grade or something. At first it didn't bother me so much. But then it started to get on my nerves. I used to try to talk to him about it, but he thought I was just being critical."

Now I understand why Rob stopped initiating sex. He clearly wasn't making her happy. Eventually he concluded she was just impossible to please—and gave up.

This actually accounts for a fair number of men who stop initiating sex. For one reason or another (and often unconsciously), they decide the situation is hopeless. See Chapter 11 for details.

Now after some encouragement Rob is back initiating. But nothing has really changed. Melissa is more frustrated than ever, and they're clearly headed for disaster again.

On the positive side, this time they're in treatment—and I'm thinking maybe I can help her find the words to tell him what she wants.

Once we can figure out exactly what that is.

The Masculine Ideal

There was energy here, a power of some kind in the way he worked. He didn't just wait for nature, he took it over in a gentle way, shaping it to his vision, making it fit what he saw in his mind.
—ROBERT JAMES WALLER,
THE BRIDGES OF MADISON COUNTY

Within the conventional script for heterosexual mating, there is an unwritten list of masculine attributes that women tend to admire. These include confidence, self-sufficiency, initiative, decisiveness, and maturity.

These are all attributes that are characteristic of leaders. Within the conventional script, men are expected to show good leadership qualities.

A woman has much more latitude in this realm. She doesn't always have to look like a leader. The conventional script gives women free rein to act needy, weak, dependent, or childish if that's what they're feeling. But for a man to display any of these qualities marks him immediately as unmasculine.

Maybe that's going to change. Maybe in the future, men and women will have equal rights to display both strength and weakness. But we're clearly not there yet.

Within the conventional script, women still have exclusive rights to act needy—both in the bedroom as well as outside of it. A man may indulge in a little neediness on special occasions. Then it can be endearing, but only because it's out of character.

Women often find it attractive when a man who's ordinarily hard and resolute suddenly shows his softer side. But softness in men can be a difficult ingredient to work with.

A touch of neediness can make a man seem more approachable, or more complex. But chronic neediness on a man's part is sure to turn most women off. Too much softness can render the whole thing unerotic.

Do you remember we talked in Chapter 3 about how sexual arousal naturally evokes childlike, regressive feelings? That's all fine in the abstract, but in male-female relationships it's chiefly women who are permitted to express such feelings.

Women are ordinarily free to indulge in pouting, baby talk, and total silliness in bed. But for men these things tend still to be taboo.

A woman can do the "daddy" thing with a man, and enjoy feeling dependent on him every once in a while. But a man can't usually do the "mommy" thing with a woman without seriously turning her off.

A man can lose himself entirely in a woman's arms for a few moments before ejaculating. He can become momentarily as helpless as a baby at the breast, and most women will find that gratifying.

But if he were to do this throughout lovemaking, she'd probably think he was being unmasculine.

Again, it's a question of balance.

The Man with No Feelings

"There's something else too," says Melissa. "Something I've never told anyone."

Whatever it is, it's making her blush. She's talking very fast, and I realize it's the first time I've ever seen her looking at all enthusiastic.

"Sometimes when I masturbate," she says, "I fantasize that I'm with some faceless man who doesn't care about me at all. He just uses my body for his own pleasure—like I'm totally *disposable*. After he's done with me, he just tosses me away."

Melissa takes a deep breath, still red from blushing.

"I don't know why, but that really turns me on."

I'm not at all surprised to hear this. For some reason, this fantasy is one I hear from a lot of women in my office these days.

Melissa assures me that in reality she'd *never* want to be with somebody like that, who didn't care about her. But this isn't about reality. This is about sex. To quote Esther Perel, "Most of us get turned on at night by the very things that we'll demonstrate against during the day."

Power is sexy, and many women tell me they get excited by the idea of surrendering to a partner who has a lot of it. The man in Melissa's fantasy doesn't care about her *at all*—which in such a fantasy is a position of tremendous power.

In their real relationship, when Rob tries too hard to please Melissa he gives her all the power.

That gives her certain advantages, of course. But it's definitely not erotic. Few straight women enjoy feeling consistently more powerful than their partners in bed.

Melissa stares at a bare spot on the wall. She's quiet for a long moment, obviously deep in thought.

"Here's another thing," she says finally. "This feeling—when I fantasize being with this faceless man to whom I'm nothing—it's kind of *liberating*. I don't understand that at all."

"Liberating?"

"Yeah, that's what's so strange. He doesn't care about me at all. I can't figure out why that's so refreshing."

"Maybe it means you don't have to care about *him*?"

"Hmm. I never thought of that."

"Sure. You can just surrender."

"That *does* sound refreshing." She thinks hard. "Just to turn off my mind and let go."

"Do you ever use this fantasy when you're with Rob?" I ask.

"I'd love to, but it doesn't work. It doesn't fit with who he is."

As I listen, it occurs to me that I still don't really *know* who Rob is. He's a bit of a cipher—a handsome well-tailored man who doesn't say much. What's behind Rob's relentless need for Melissa's approval in bed?

"I think some of it might be from his father," says Melissa. "I never knew Rob's father—he died a few years before we met—but everyone seems to have been afraid of him. He had a bad temper, he drank too much, and I think he may have hit Rob's mother."

"Were Rob and his mother close?"

"Yes, they still are. She's had a hard life. I think Rob feels protective of her."

This is a very familiar story—one I hear several times a year. A son has a father whom he hates so much that rather than identifying with him, he *dis-identifies* with him. He tries to make sure he's as little like his father as possible.

If the father is domineering, the son becomes as un-domineering as he can. The son grows up to be a man who's too nice, too deferential, and can't express any raw male passion because he's afraid of being too much like his father.

"What do you think I should do?" she asks.

My first thought is that I'd like to have a discussion about this with Rob. But there'll be time for that later. Melissa wants something she can do right now that might be helpful.

"Have you ever thought of sharing this fantasy of yours with him?" I ask.

"No," she says. "But I'll do it, if you think it might help."

"It's a bit of a gamble," I tell her. "But sometimes a fantasy is worth a thousand words."

She says she'll give it a try.

One Week Later

The next week when I meet Rob and Melissa in the waiting room, he has his hands out of his pockets, and she's not on her phone for once. I take all this as a good sign.

"How are things going?" I ask.

"A little better," Rob says. "I think Melissa finally got what she wanted."

She nods, smiling broadly. "Definitely."

"What did he do?" I ask.

"He finally took charge. Nothing too kinky. He just did me without all that solicitude. I didn't know he had it in him."

"What do you think helped?"

"I told him about my fantasy," she says.

Rob stands and takes off his suit jacket, then sits back down again.

"I realized I'd been holding back on her because I didn't want to seem, well, *domineering*. Melissa made me see there's a difference between being domineering and being *dominant*."

"That's an important distinction," I say. "A lot of men never figure that out."

"My father was a tyrant. I swore to myself I'd never be like that." Rob looks at me earnestly.

"My mother said it made her happy that I was so different. My aunts too. That made me feel good, but it also made me anxious—especially when I became a teenager and realized I had the same hard lust toward women that I imagined my father had. I didn't know what to do with that, so I guess I just buried it."

"A lot of men bury that part of themselves," I tell him. "Especially with their wives."

Men, Women, and Pleasure

There's been a major shake-up in our sexual culture in the last half century, and I think most men still haven't recovered from it.

Kinsey's surveys of women in the 1950s showed clearly what everyone had denied for centuries: that many women were indeed interested in sex. Then along came Masters and Johnson, with their direct observations of men and women masturbating and having sex in the laboratory—and all of a sudden everyone knew about women's multiple orgasms and their greater capacity for sustained arousal.

Masters and Johnson were all about shifting from performance to pleasure. It *was* the sixties, after all. Birth control pills moved the conversation even further.

In the blink of an eye, sexual pleasure became a thing.

Once that happened, it suddenly became obvious that we men were in over our heads.

Most women tend to know instinctively how to enjoy pure physical pleasure—whether at the nail salon, the spa, or just appreciating beautiful things. Most men not so much.

I don't know how much of this is culture and how much biology, but most men tend to avoid pure pleasure just as we tended to throw off our mothers' embraces when we were boys. For all I know, these two things may be related.

Today it's largely women who think seriously about erotic pleasure. At the sex therapy meetings I attend, the ratio of women to men is usually at least six to one.

My colleague Betty Dodson once made a video entitled *Orgasmic Women: 13 Selfloving Divas*—a warm, admiring montage of thirteen women, each demonstrating her favorite masturbation techniques on camera. As of this writing, it's available on her website and on Amazon.

No one outside the gay male community celebrates male sexual pleasure that way—purely, just for its own sake. If you're a woman who loves to masturbate, you're a self-loving diva. For a heterosexual man, it's not considered worthy of admiration.

Male sexual pleasure is still out there somewhere in the shadows.

"Nonsense," say my female colleagues. "It's *always* been about men's pleasure. Their leering looks on the street. Their constant objectification of women's bodies. Their insistent need to penetrate and get off. We women are just trying to claim some space for ourselves."

Point taken. And I know many women have trouble allowing themselves sexual pleasure as well. But the conventional script for heterosexual mating has always been more concerned with a man's adequacy in bed than with how much he's really enjoying the experience.

What Not to Talk About at a Sex Therapy Conference

The erotic delight that a woman might feel from her own beauty has its counterpart in a man's admiration of his own erect penis. Unfortunately for straight men, few women are really that interested in penises—except as a barometer of how much a partner desires them, or for stimulation during intercourse.

In the progressive sex circles where I travel, penises tend to get associated with the patriarchy, and with men's feelings of sexual entitlement. There's no better way to lose an audience at a sex therapy meeting than to bring up the subject of men's erections. You could go to these meetings for years and never know there was such a thing as a penis.

Objects like columns or tall towers that look like erect penises have long symbolized patriarchal authority. This is unfortunate, since in reality men can't control their erections any more than they can control any other involuntary body function.

Erections are the most vulnerable part of a man's sexual response—for both medical and psychological reasons. Loss of hardness is often a psychological catastrophe for a man.

No one knows exactly why. I think it's primarily because of the archaic way we associate erections with masculinity. Most men feel lost without this physical emblem of their manhood.

Within the conventional script, masculinity is never a given. It has to be earned, and it can easily be lost or taken away. Often a man who's been unable to get hard in bed with a partner will tell me, "I don't feel like a man anymore."

Maybe in a less patriarchal society this wouldn't be so big a deal. I don't know. All I know is we're definitely not there yet.

The conventional script still tends to see manhood as about "doing," as we've discussed. In most men's minds, an erection is a thing you *do* something with. If you're not hard, it's as if you're at the job site without your tools.

Of course this is nonsense. Your bedroom is not a job site, and you *can* do a lot in bed without an erection. But most men feel otherwise.

For most men, making love while worrying about staying hard is a bit like trying to enjoy a movie while worrying about whether the projector is going to work. You're not going to be able to enjoy the movie very much.

After a while, you're not going to want to go back to that theater either. Worrying about erections is probably the most common reason men avoid sex.

~~

When all's said and done, what's the main reason a man needs to get hard?

Is it so he can have intercourse? No, that's too practical.

The main reason a man needs to get hard is so he won't have to worry about getting hard.

Having an erection is no guarantee that he'll enjoy himself. But if he *doesn't* have one, there's not much chance he'll remember the experience fondly.

Katherine and Rich

Katherine is an accomplished fifty-something professional woman with two grown children. She and her husband, Rich, have sex once a week, and she says it's boring her to tears.

According to Katherine, it's pretty much the same thing every time. They make out a little, and then she strokes his penis to get him hard.

"Does he like that?" I ask.

"I never really asked him. I assume he does."

"Do *you* like it?"

"I guess it's okay."

There's a pause, then she scrunches up her nose. "Actually, not really."

"Yeah. Sounds like a chore. Yuck."

She giggles.

Katherine isn't alone in feeling this way. Most women say it's not terribly erotic having to stroke your husband's penis to get it hard.

But the alternative—waiting around for him to get hard on his own—isn't usually much better. In the old days we used to recommend that couples just try to ignore the state of the man's erection and instead focus on other things. But that's an advanced technique, and few people were capable of it. These days most couples roll their eyes if I even suggest it.

I find it's often an act of mercy for the man to take Viagra or some other PDE5 inhibitor medication. They don't always work—especially if his erection problems are more advanced, or their emotional problems are more serious. But for many couples, medication just makes it easier to get things going in an erotic direction.

Rich's urologist prescribes Viagra, and it works like a charm.

"I wish I'd done this years ago," he tells Katherine a few weeks later in my office. "I used to hate it when you had to stroke me to get me hard. I always worried it wasn't going to work."

Many months later when they have their sexual groove back, Rich lets me show him some simple techniques for enhancing his erotic focus.

"Don't worry about Katherine," I tell him. "Just attend to your own arousal."

"Won't she feel ignored?"

"Most likely she'll find it liberating—not having to worry about *you.*"

"What if I *don't* feel aroused?"

"Just notice that. Don't get too involved with it. See what the next moment brings."

Rich tries this technique, and likes it. He learns that arousal comes in its own time, if you just stay out of its way.

But Rich says he still can't really relax during sex unless he's taken his Viagra. Even though he knows he'll eventually get hard, it's just too stressful having to wait.

Maybe in the future we'll have evolved to where middle-aged men can enjoy lovemaking without having to worry about their erections. But I'm not holding my breath.

Viagra for a man like Rich can be the equivalent of good lubricant for a middle-aged woman: a reasonable accommodation to the reality that you're not a teenager anymore. And an acknowledgment that even the wisest and most mature among us will inevitably be a bit impatient in bed.

~~

The conventional script is still rather unyielding in its insistence on male performance—both inside and outside the bedroom. Just as it's still harsh in its demands for female beauty.

No one knows how much of this script is encoded in our DNA and how much is culturally transmitted. It's likely that culture amplifies something that's already there.

Our culture is changing. Relationships today tend to be more egalitarian, and many married women now earn more than their husbands. But I haven't seen much change yet in people's expectations of male performance—sexual or otherwise.

Straight women in my office still seem to crave displays of male leadership, confidence, and drive. And dominant men still get lots of female attention, while submissive ones often can't get a date.

We'll see if any of this changes in the future, as traditional gender lines become more blurred. I think it may be awhile though before men truly feel comfortable receiving erotic pleasure for its own sake. And a long time before most men can think clearly about their own erotic pleasure without also worrying about how well they're performing.

The Mysteries of Intercourse

While foreplay (as its name suggests) connotes play, intercourse is seen by most people as serious business. No one seems to think of intercourse as play.

This can lead to all sorts of problems.

"Lord of Peace . . .
You alone unite opposites, and bring them together in peace, and in great love."
—RABBI NACHMAN OF BRESLOV

Vagina Dentata

For some reason, just about all male sexual dysfunctions get worse in the presence of a willing vagina. I don't know why. It's a deep mystery, which to my knowledge no one has ever been able to solve.

One man may stay perfectly hard during foreplay, but put his penis anywhere near her vagina and he'll immediately go soft.

Another man might tolerate all kinds of physical stimulation without climaxing, but the minute his penis goes into her vagina he won't be able to hold back his orgasm.

And yet another may be able to climax over and over again in bed with his partner—anywhere except inside her.

Something about the vagina just seems to get guys where they live.

In Freud's time, one heard about male fantasies of *vagina dentata*—the vagina with teeth.

Some men really do seem to be afraid of putting their penis inside a partner's body, where they can't see it.

Is it safe in there? How does he know for sure she'll return it to him intact?

The reality, of course, is that a woman is in much more danger from a man's penis than he might be from her vagina. But many men still get spooked by women's genitals, whether they're conscious of this or not.

I've sometimes had to explain to a particularly squeamish man that no, the vagina is not an internal organ. It's not actually blood and guts. Once men understand that their partner's vagina is really more like her mouth—just an extension of the outside, folded in—they often calm down about it.

Some men are particularly haunted by the fear of getting their partner pregnant. I remember once speaking to a group of women about how men are afraid of their partners' vaginas. At one point an extremely pregnant woman in the front row shouted, "*They should be!*"

Even with state-of-the-art contraception, some men have an exaggerated dread that if their penis falls into the vagina their life might spin out of control.

My guess though is that fears of pregnancy and bodily injury account for only a small percent of the huge number of straight men who lose sexual function at the moment of penetration. I think for the majority of these men it's something more subtle.

Most good heterosexual foreplay dramatizes the man's hunger for his partner's body. And most straight women enjoy the fact that their male partners are hungry for them. (Some women say they enjoy this more than anything else.)

It's common for a straight woman to like that her body has within it the capacity to give a man exactly what he wants. He is the hungry baby, and she is the all-giving mother—ready to supply him with her inner riches.

Once it's clear she's interested in having intercourse, the atmosphere changes. Now she wants something from *him*. He imagines her vagina opening for him like a hungry mouth. For many men, this is an anxious moment—even though they know this mouth has no teeth in it.

Unconsciously, many men feel they lack sufficient inner resources to satisfy a partner. Men aren't accustomed to being the providers of physical nourishment. It makes them nervous.

A woman's need can seem enormous—too much for him. He worries she'll be ravenous and want more than he has to give.

Viewed this way, it's no surprise that many men lose sexual function the moment intercourse appears on the menu. Given the depth of feeling that can be involved, it's remarkable that intercourse so often proceeds without a hitch.

The Penis and the Breast

Intercourse can be joyful, but it's not typically carefree. Foreplay can be a bit lighthearted. Hey, it's even called "play." But no one seems to think of intercourse as play.

Once penetration happens, people tend to lose whatever sense of humor they might have started out with when they first decided to get naked together.

As with so much else in erotic life, the explanation for this may lie in childhood.

The original act of penetration is the mother's nipple in the infant's mouth. Whatever loving playfulness might have been going on between a mother and her baby, once actual nursing commences it's no longer playful.

Nursing a baby doesn't just involve the nipple, of course. At its best, it's full-on skin to skin.

Pleasure and seriousness are fused in a way that doesn't occur again except during great sex.

The wish to possess the mother, like the wish to be nourished by her, is never a casual impulse. It's initially a matter of life and death, since infants who have no one to bond with don't survive.

The mother-infant bond is the first experience of that childlike possessiveness we talked so much about in Part I—"*I am my beloved's, and my beloved is mine.*"

Intercourse can be the quintessential adult expression of that same possessive impulse. There's no other sexual act that marks a partner so clearly as "mine."

Finally there's the obvious fact that penis-vagina intercourse can result in a baby. On a human level this remains a deep mystery, no matter how much we understand the science involved.

From a sex therapy perspective, intercourse *should* feel mysterious. Even astonishing. That's part of what makes it erotic. But people vary in how much astonishment they're able to bear.

Most straight people see intercourse as the only really "grown-up" way to have sex, and they feel like failures if for whatever reason intercourse isn't working out for them.

Gay and lesbian couples, operating largely outside the conventional script, aren't as affected by this kind of symbolism. Among many LGBT folks, whether or not you choose to do some kind of penetration depends more on whether it's something you actually enjoy.

Some gay male couples love anal intercourse and do it every chance they get. Many others don't like it at all. Some lesbians want something inside them—whether it's a toy, a strap-on, or a partner's fingers—and some don't particularly care for it.

For straight people though, if you're not having intercourse at least some of the time it usually feels like there's something wrong.

Simply taking a break from the goal of achieving intercourse can help with a substantial number of sex problems. But for most people that's easier said than done—especially when all you can think of is that everyone else is having intercourse and you're not.

Back to the Clitoris

A woman's vagina is designed to stroke a man's penis to orgasm, so most straight men find intercourse very rewarding. But women vary widely in how much they enjoy it.

Some women consider penis-vagina intercourse to be one of life's greatest pleasures, while some equally normal women get very little from it and have trouble understanding what all the fuss is about.

For some it's an acquired taste. Others say they never understood the appeal until they finally had a partner who knew how to do it well.

If you're a woman who loves intercourse, you may value the deep connection you feel while "containing" your partner's penis. Or the sense of possessing him completely. But most of the actual *physical* stimulation you feel probably comes from indirect stimulation of your clitoris.

As we discussed in Chapter 6, most of your clitoris is deep inside where you can't see it. Much of your "inner clitoris," in fact, is wrapped tightly around your vagina. It's often worth experimenting to find what angles of penetration stroke your inner clitoris the best. This might be different with one partner than with another, since men's shapes and angles vary.

You might find that to really enjoy intercourse you need some stimulation of your "outer clitoris" as well. Hands and fingers—either yours or your partner's—can serve nicely, and some sex positions are better than others for allowing hands and fingers full access during penetration.

Or you can do what's called "coital alignment technique": taking his penis deep inside you, until your outer clitoris sits snugly in that little niche just above the base of his penis.

Now when he thrusts up high inside you, he's stroking your outer clitoris much more directly. You can also grind up against *him*, putting your outer clitoris exactly where you want it and controlling the action yourself.

That's a good idea if you're trying to climax, since only you know what rhythms you might need moment to moment in order to get there.

Pain and Numbness

Most women have had intercourse-related pain at some point in their lives. But a sizable number of women *consistently* have pain during or after penetrative sex.

Some women find it hurts whenever a partner's penis (or anything else) touches the entrance to their vagina. Others tend to tense their pelvic muscles involuntarily, which can make penetration painful or impossible. There are other medical causes as well.

If your regular gynecologist doesn't have the answer, it's best to go directly to someone who specializes in this kind of problem. No, it's not in your head.

A surprising number of women keep having intercourse even when it hurts. So a partner shouldn't assume she's not in pain just because she doesn't complain about it. When in doubt, just ask.

Many women feel emotionally or physically *numb* during penetrative sex. Intercourse puts them in a kind of dissociative state where they're not really sure what they feel.

Some don't even know it's happening. Others have just always experienced intercourse this way, and aren't aware there's anything wrong.

Sometimes it's because of anxiety, or feeling angry at a partner, or some other troublesome emotion. But for many women it's due to trauma in their past—most often the trauma of having been sexually molested, assaulted, or coerced into sex.*

Like physical pain during intercourse, a feeling of numbness or emotional confusion should be respected as a sign that you've gone beyond the limit of what feels good, and that you should stop what you're doing.

If you find yourself dissociating, don't just go through the motions. If you can summon the courage, tell your partner what's really going on. This can help immeasurably. Silence tends to breed shame and disconnection. Breaking the silence gives you the opportunity to connect again.

If you're going to have intercourse, make sure the conditions are right. Don't do if it hurts, or if it makes you feel numb or confused. Don't just do it to get it over with, or because you can't think of any other way to end the evening. And *definitely* don't do it if your partner is making you uncomfortable.

Remember, the only good reason to have intercourse is because you want to.

Why You Should Never Hurry Penetration

Intercourse can be intensely exciting. But it can also get very boring—especially if you weren't that aroused to begin with.

Many straight couples make the mistake of thinking that once they're hard and wet enough that they *can* do it, that means they *should*. They hurry to check it off the list before they're really excited enough.

I tell my patients to imagine sexual arousal on a scale from 0 to 100—like a speedometer that measures your *total* turn-on: mental, physical, everything.

---

* Coercion can take many forms, such as submitting to intercourse because you're too intoxicated to fully resist, being afraid your partner will get angry if you say no, or just deciding to get it over with so he'll let you go home. Any situation where you don't feel fully free to choose constitutes coercion.

Here's how I tend to think of this:

0.	Not aroused
20.	Becoming aroused
40.	Fully aroused
60.	Intensely aroused
80.	Very intensely aroused
100.	Theoretical limit of human arousability

If you're young and healthy, you probably only need an arousal level of 20 or so to get hard or wet. But sex at a 20 isn't usually that exciting.

Better to lose a few more IQ points first. Ideally you should save penetration until you're at least at an arousal level of 40. Fully aroused.

Wait until you're really hungry for it. Some playful teasing beforehand can heighten the drama and make intercourse more exciting.

Instead of just going in right away, maybe have him dab some lubricant on the head of his penis and use it like a paintbrush across your vulva—up and down, back and forth, then round and round the opening of your vagina until you both find it hard to resist taking the plunge.

Sex on a Stopwatch

Some men need very little stimulation to get off. That's just how they're wired. Add the ordinary male tendency to freak out around intercourse and many such men end up ejaculating within seconds of penetration.

Most men with this problem try to delay orgasm by keeping their arousal below thirty. But that's like intentionally trying to have bad sex.

My patient Clara has this to say about sex with her husband, Chris: "I don't really mind Chris coming so quickly inside me," she said. "Intercourse has never been especially my thing. What really upsets me is that all he focuses on is not ejaculating. It's as if I'm not even there."

Clara and Chris have already been to a sex therapist, who taught them to do what's called "stop-start"—where they stop moving every time he feels an orgasm coming on. Stop-start can be a wonderful technique if a man is only slightly premature. But for someone like Chris who has a really low orgasm threshold, the only way to make stop-start work is for Clara to lie very still and make sure she doesn't moan. Not much fun.

There *is* another way, but it involves medication. All of the so-called serotonin reuptake inhibitors (SRIs)—Prozac, Zoloft the whole bunch—tend to help men get and stay more excited without ejaculating. The FDA has never approved any of them for this use, but doctors are free to prescribe any medication "off-label" as long as the patient gives appropriate informed consent.

I've treated many men for premature ejaculation with SRIs. They've been some of my most grateful patients.

A lot though depends on the quality of your relationship. If your partner accepts you just as you are, but you'd really like to be able to have hotter sex without having to shut down your arousal, then medication might be a reasonable option.

But sometimes a man may just have a very critical partner, and his prematurity makes him an easy target for her criticism. In that situation, I don't love the idea of his taking a drug to make her happy. It usually doesn't work.

Remember: Acceptance. *Vitamin A.*

If your partner is really that unhappy with you, then you really might just be better off finding another partner.

Higher Love

For most people, the upper levels of arousal—60 or above on my scale—don't happen so often. That's perfectly okay. But there are some people who spend their lives in pursuit of the higher peaks. Sexual intensity is what they love best. That's just who they are.

It's like skiing. Many people love to ski. But only a few individuals take helicopters to really edgy, out-of-the-way places where the skiing is truly spectacular.

A lot of sex books are written by such people. That's understandable, but it's not much help to the rest of us who just want to get down the mountain with good form and not get hurt.

High-intensity arousal is also more likely to happen *outside* of a committed relationship. To quote the late Jack Morin, "We are the most intensely excited when we are a little off-balance, uncertain, poised on the perilous edge between ecstasy and disaster."

That kind of emotional intensity is rarely sustainable with someone with whom you share a mortgage.

My feeling is that as long as you get *fully aroused* together—40 or so on my scale—you've got all you really need. Most erotically happy couples stay consistently around 40, and still have perfectly great sex.

But let's say you yearn to scale the higher peaks. Are there any good ways to achieve this that don't require you to ruin your life?

The best way I know of is simply to assess your level of arousal in the moment—then ask yourself, "What might I do to get a little higher than I am right now?"

In general this is best achieved by learning to enhance your erotic focus—something we started talking about in Chapter 6.

Pay attention to your breath. Take time to fully notice the sensations in your body. Maybe there's somewhere else you're yearning to touch your partner. Or somewhere else you're yearning to be touched. These things can become much clearer once you start really paying attention.

Getting to 80 is impressive. And these days there's no shortage of experts eager to show you how to do it. So go ahead and sign up for that Tantra class if you like.

But don't worry if you and your partner just tend to cruise at a 40 most of the time. If you do that the right way on a steady basis, that's plenty enough to fuel an erotic relationship for a lifetime—as we'll see in Part III.

Sex-Knots

For many straight couples, the most challenging thing about intercourse is that it requires the man to have an erection.

Loss of an erection is extremely stressful for a man. Unfortunately, it can be stressful for his partner too. If a man loses hardness repeatedly, a partner can start to worry that maybe he doesn't desire them. As you know, that's very bad.

Now throw in the fact that each partner's sexual self has the maturity of a two-year-old at best, and it's easy to see how all hell might quickly break loose in bed.

Hal and Deborah have been seeing each other for a few months. They've been having a lot of sex—partly out of desire for each other, and partly (like all new couples) just for reassurance that everything's still okay. He's lost his erection a few times with her, which worries him because he never knows when that's going to happen.

Now Hal and Deborah are going to spend a weekend at a beautiful resort. Hal wants this to be a memorable trip. He's eager to have a lot of sex with Deborah, but he also realizes the stakes are somewhat higher.

It's Friday evening and they've just arrived at the resort. They go out for a nice romantic dinner together. Then they head up to bed—both feeling a little nervous.

Here's what can happen next:

Hal worries about getting hard. Since if he loses it now, it's going to be a bad start to the weekend.

This (naturally) interferes with his ability to get hard. Because his sexual self, being naturally childish, has decided the pressure is too much and that now would be a good time to ruin everything.

This makes him worry even more. Which of course *seriously* interferes with his ability to get hard.

Of course, the presence of another person in bed makes things even more complicated:

Deborah worries that Hal might not be that attracted to her. Because otherwise he'd be hard, right?

She gets upset.

This makes *him* upset, and even less likely to get hard. His sexual self, having by now concluded that the situation is hopeless, has decided to shut down permanently for the night.

Now she's *sure* he's not attracted to her.

And so on, and so on.

～～

I've come to refer to this kind of a situations as a "sex-knot." Once you find yourself in a sex-knot, it's difficult to avoid pulling the knot tighter—even if you don't mean to.

Not all sex-knots require two people. But it takes two to tie the really gnarly ones.

Sex-knots are the main reason sexual problems can be so difficult to fix.

A good sex therapist could easily show you how to untie a knot like this. But sex therapists are hard to find in most parts of the world, and they tend to be expensive.

So in the next couple of chapters I'm going to show you how to untie some of the most common sex-knots on your own. I've also included a more extensive guide at the back of this book. Go have a look now if you want. I'll wait.

~~~

To solve Hal and Deborah's sex-knot, it's important to keep in mind that penises are very good at *being*—but they get pressured into *doing* in order to satisfy men's ideals of masculinity and their partners' need to feel desirable.

Hal's penis is never going to function well under this kind of pressure. It's too emotionally immature, and way too easily overwhelmed.

Instead, when Hal and Deborah first get into bed, maybe he could just tell her he's feeling nervous. A good partner will understand that an intimate communication like this took courage.

Maybe Deborah will respond by telling him she feels nervous too.

With any luck, Hal will feel understood and accepted (remember, vitamin A)—which for most people is a wonderfully happy feeling and a great relief. Hal's penis will then express this happy feeling in the only language it knows.

When this happens, though, Hal might want to avoid the temptation to *do* something with his erection immediately.

It's often better, if only for a moment, to just let it *be*.

Then, of Course, There's *Condoms*

Using a condom isn't as simple as you'd think. A surprising number of men can't seem to keep an erection while putting one on.

To use a condom the right way, a man needs to know how genuinely aroused he is. An arousal of twenty represents the bare minimum. If you start putting on a condom when you're only at a twenty, it's going to be very easy to slip down to a fifteen and lose your erection before you get the thing on.

Best to wait to put on a condom until you're at a solid forty. Then even if you lose a lot of points while putting it on, you'll still be okay.

It's also crucially important not to hurry to penetrate once you get the condom on. Hurrying penetration is always a bad idea, as you know. With a condom on, it's worse.

All sorts of things can happen during penetration. A random worry about something irrelevant. A little trouble penetrating because your partner isn't relaxed enough. A few moments' delay to get the geometry right. Any of these things can make you lose points.

Your sexual self doesn't much like goals—even pleasurable ones. So instead of penetrating right away after putting on the condom, it's much better to hit "rewind" and go back to whatever kind of foreplay you were doing that got you to a forty in the first place.

Then when you're up around forty again, go ahead and penetrate if you both feel ready.

Remember to take your time though. You didn't come all this way to waste it on bad sex.

Makes sense? Good. This is one place where learning to tune in to your arousal can literally save your life.

Getting Practical:
Intercourse, Outercourse, and "Lazy Sex"

Masters and Johnson invented modern sex therapy, and for several years they were the only sex therapists in the world. For a while in the 1960s, if you wanted help for a sexual problem, your only option was to spend two weeks at the Masters and Johnson clinic in St. Louis.

Treatment would typically begin with your being told to stop having intercourse. This made good sense, since intercourse is where most couples get into trouble.

The mutual friction of penetrative sex would seem to ensure mutuality in lovemaking, but often it doesn't. Once you move beyond the idea that real sex has to involve some kind of penetration, you're freer to focus on genuine arousal. As Masters and Johnson knew, "outercourse" can sometimes be just the thing to restore a couple's erotic energy.

Once you get past the idea that you're obligated to do intercourse, it's not such a big step to give up the notion that lovemaking has to be mutual every time.

The conventional script holds that once you're in a partnership, you're no longer allowed to touch your own genitals in bed. But that's silly.

I see many couples where one partner wants sex a lot more than the other. Under such circumstances, the idea of mutuality can be tyrannical. Most people in relationships still masturbate. Why not do it in bed with your partner where it's warm and cozy?

On occasions when you really want to have sex but your partner doesn't, I usually recommend the following:

Give yourself an orgasm with your own hand (or a vibrator) while your partner rubs up against you in bed—or holds you in his or her arms. If you do this fully naked, with lots of deep kissing and skin-on-skin contact, it can have almost all the ingredients of conventional lovemaking without the need for penetration.

A patient of mine once dubbed this kind of thing "lazy sex." Lazy sex is ideal for new parents, for people on different sleep schedules, or once in a while just for the heck of it. All you need is to get over the idea that sex has to be mutual every time.

Penetrative sex is unique in that you have to be mindful of how the two of you actually fit together. Penises protrude at various angles, and they come in all sizes. Sometimes the geometric fit between two people seems ideal, and sometimes not.

Changing positions can help, and most couples eventually settle on a few favorite positions where they fit together best. Still, it sometimes happens that for one reason or another a couple is just not cut out for great penetrative sex. One woman might need twenty minutes of serious pounding in order to climax, while her male partner may come in a matter of seconds. Other women whose husbands have very large penises can find intercourse painful if it lasts more than a few minutes.

When this happens, you may want to consider having "outercourse" rather than intercourse as your "main course." As my fellow sex-writer Ian Kerner says, sometimes it can be a good idea to promote foreplay to "core-play."

Sure, you can finish off with intercourse if the symbolism is important to you, or if you like the feeling of mutuality. Just make sure it's real mutuality, and that you're not forcing the situation in order to satisfy an ideal of what sex should be like.

Remember, sex should be easy. Many sexually happy men pull out after ten minutes of great penetrative sex and finish themselves off by hand, because it's easier for them to come that way. And many erotically satisfied women prefer to finish themselves off with a vibrator while their partner presses up against them and kisses their hair.

10

Why Women Lose Interest in Sex

Most women are built not to want sex unless certain specific conditions are met.

That's true for most men too, of course. But most women's conditions tend to be more exacting.

"I think about sex a lot. It is on my mind the first thing in the morning, and it is invariably the last thing I think about at night. Every morning I get up and say to myself that today I will have sex with my husband; I will do it. By noon I can feel my resolve waning, and by evening I am feeling so stressed that sex is out of the question."
—"ANNA," QUOTED IN KATHRYN HALL,
RECLAIMING YOUR SEXUAL SELF

Marnie and Tom met in college, and after first sleeping together they almost never slept apart. When people asked them the secret to their happy marriage, they'd always say it was that they found each other physically irresistible.

Tom was usually the one to initiate sex. But if Tom showed Marnie the right kind of desire, she was always easily aroused.

Marnie had expected she might feel less interested in sex after having a baby. But when that actually happened she was shocked at how dramatic the change really was. Many months after delivering their first child, sex was still the farthest thing from her mind.

For the first time in her life, sex with Tom felt like a chore.

Marnie could still get aroused and have a climax. Afterward she'd think, "That wasn't so bad. We should do that more often." But she still rarely felt like it.

Sex just seemed an unnecessary bother. If only Tom felt the same way, Marnie thought, then everything would be perfect.

Something was seriously off-kilter.

The Mysteries of Desire

Masters and Johnson never attempted to study sexual desire. That may have been good judgment on their part, since it's a confusing subject.

Masters and Johnson limited their field of study to what they called the "sex response cycle," which was all about getting more blood flow to the genitals and preparing for orgasm. Desire never really figured into it.

But the individuals and couples who'd volunteered for Masters and Johnson's original sex studies weren't ordinary people. Most people—especially most women—won't take their clothes off and mate with a near stranger during their lunch hour for the sake of science, as many of Masters and Johnson's subjects did.

Helen Kaplan understood there was something missing from the Masters and Johnson model. Her solution was to tack on something called "desire" at the beginning of Masters and Johnson's "sex response cycle."

The idea had a kind of intuitive appeal. After all, you obviously need *something* to get sex going. But there never was really much science behind it.

Back when sexologists were mostly male, desire used to be thought of as some kind of hydraulic pressure in the body—like the pressure most young men feel when they need to ejaculate.

But the hydraulic model doesn't fit the facts of most women's desire. Women tend to need a good *reason* to have sex. Otherwise, most women can go for a long time without feeling desire.

Like the screen-saver program on an old-fashioned desktop computer, a woman's system will often stay in "sleep mode" until someone moves the mouse.

There are also lots of reasons a woman might *not* want to have sex.

A list of all these could easily fill several books.

Stress and exhaustion would certainly top most modern women's list. Then there's hating your body; feeling angry, depressed, or worried; painful intercourse; too much pressure to have an orgasm; bad sex in general; or any combination of the above.

Trauma from your past can make you not want to have sex— sometimes years or decades later, when you least expect it. So can being abused or mistreated by your current partner. Or knowing there's no future in the relationship, but not being quite ready to leave.

These are all quite rational reasons a woman might not want to have sex. There are of course many others—all of them quite rational.

In addition, there's one big *irrational* reason:

Worrying that there's something wrong with you for not feeling desire.

This thought itself can knock out a woman's sexual desire very quickly.

Many women I see in the office are always on the verge of

thinking there's something wrong with them. I don't know why this is. But it's everywhere, and it causes a lot of trouble.

When a woman who's prone to this kind of thinking loses desire, it often leads immediately to the following sex-knot:

> **You have no desire for sex.**
>
> **You think, "There must be something wrong with me."**
>
> **Now you *definitely* have no desire for sex.**

Women in my office vary tremendously in how they feel about losing desire. Some married women seem strangely not to care— despite the frustration of a partner who has no other possible sexual outlet except masturbation or infidelity.

I think many women try not to reflect on their loss of desire because it just makes them worry there's something wrong with them.

That thought is never far from a lot of women's minds.

What Not to Do When You've Lost Desire

Some women who've lost desire will keep having sex with their partner out of a sense of responsibility—or just to keep the peace. This is seldom a good idea.

Your sexual self has no idea what the word "responsibility" even means. All your sexual self knows is that it's being forced to do something it doesn't want to do.

It doesn't like that one bit, of course. So what happens next is no surprise:

> **You lose desire.**
>
> **Sex begins to feel like an obligation.**
>
> **Now you *really* lose desire.**

Obligation sex also creates the problem of trying to hide from your partner the fact that you're just not that into it. Eventually you might find yourself faking excitement—which to your sexual self is like when children see adults being extra nice to people they dislike.

If you fake excitement often enough, your sexual self will lose all faith in you.

Most low-desire women eventually realize that obligation sex isn't the answer. But then there's still the problem of what to do with a partner who's still interested.

Under the circumstances, many women start avoiding anything that might turn their partner on. No sexy underwear. No lingering kisses. Nothing that might put them in the uncomfortable position of having to say no.

It's easy to see where this might lead:

You have no desire.

You worry that if your partner gets turned on, they'll get frustrated and angry.

So you shut yourself down sexually.

Now you *totally* have no desire.

You might even start staying up later and later at night, hoping your partner will be asleep by the time you get to bed. Some couples' bedtime rituals become an intricate dance around the question of whether they're going to wind up in bed awake together or not.

Loss of sexual desire can start out quite innocently and understandably, and then turn into something bigger that involves your whole attitude toward lovemaking.

By the time most women who've lost desire come to see me in

the office, their feelings about sex have shifted radically—as follows:

Situation	Previous Feelings	New Feelings
Thinking about having sex	Anticipation	Dread
After having sex	Satisfaction	Relief
Partner not in the mood	Disappointment	Relief

To state the obvious, these "new feelings" are definitely not erotic. Quite the opposite. Sometimes they're not even so new.

A thousand sex-knots can spring from this kind of soil.

Life in an Asexual Universe

Things have gotten worse now since Marnie had her second child. After feeding and caring for two young children all day long, by nightfall the only thing Marnie wants is for no one to touch her body until the morning.

Tom still often feels turned on lying in bed next to her. But now Marnie is only willing to have sex with Tom every couple of weeks, at best. She only does it to pacify him.

Marnie sees other women enjoying men's erotic attention, and she can remember feeling that way. But now she lives in a strange alternate universe where everyone else but Marnie speaks the language of eroticism—a language she's somehow lost the ability to understand.

When I first meet Marnie and Tom in the office, it's been three years since their youngest child was born. "What would you like to accomplish here?" I ask them after we've taken care of the preliminaries.

"I want to feel desire again," Marnie says.

"I'd love that," says Tom. "But I'd love it even more if Marnie didn't avoid me all the time."

Marnie looks surprised. "You never said anything about me avoiding you."

"Sure," says Tom. "You never change your clothes in front of me anymore. You never wear anything nice to bed. You seem to be doing everything you can to keep me away."

"I thought I was being considerate. I didn't want you to get excited."

Tom smiles. "I *like* being excited. Don't you know that?"

"But if I'm *not* excited—" she asks. "Isn't that disappointing?"

Tom thinks for a moment. "Sure it is. But feeling like you're avoiding me is worse."

"I didn't know that," she says.

I suggest to Marnie that trying to hide her sexiness might not be so helpful for her own desire either. She agrees that makes a lot of sense.

Then I explain to Marnie about the other two major sex-knots that stifle desire: The one where you feel there's something wrong with you, and the one where you do sex out of obligation.

All of a sudden it doesn't seem such a mystery to her that sex has come to feel like such a burden.

"So what can we do about this?" she asks me.

Be Here Now

My guess is that Marnie's wish for sex has collapsed under the weight of her physical exhaustion and a few major sex-knots. There are probably other biological factors too, and she seems depressed as well. But let's see if we can untie those sex-knots first.

Most people need acceptance more than they need sex. Turn up the acceptance, and things will usually improve.

I weigh my words carefully.

"The first and most important thing," I tell her, "is just to accept that as of right now you have no interest in sex."

She raises an eyebrow and looks at me sideways. "Just *accept* it?"

"Sure. Sex is all about acceptance."

She scowls. "That sounds like giving up," she says.

"Not at all," I tell her. "You're spending way too much energy worrying about sex. Why not use that energy more constructively?"

"How?" she asks.

"Every once in a while, a few times a day if you can, just take a long moment to focus on exactly what you *are* feeling—rather than how you *wish* you could feel."

"You mean like meditating?"

"It doesn't have to be meditating. It could be anything at all—walking, doing the dishes, even eating a snack—as long as you're in the moment. Maybe just sit and pay attention to your own breathing."

"That actually sounds nice. I'll try it. But what about with Tom?"

I ponder the question for a moment. There are some standard methods in sex therapy, which we'll discuss later. But with couples like Marnie and Tom, I usually prefer to customize.

"I'd like the two of you to spend some time naked in bed together—but not to have sex. Each of you should just pay attention to your breath and your body."

Marnie looks questioningly at Tom.

"Sounds good to me," he says.

"Will we be touching?" Marnie asks.

Hmmm, I think to myself. The standard methods call for lots of touching. But the standard methods weren't intended for young mothers.

Marnie is getting touched all day by her kids. I think she really needs to be left alone.

"You're overtouched already," I tell her. "For now, just have the experience of feeling safe and welcomed by Tom without having to be touched. You can talk if you want, but no touching."

"What if Tom gets excited?"

"I told you already," says Tom. "I *like* being excited. It's not a painful thing for me."

Tom seems to really "get" the idea of nondemand arousal. I wonder where he learned that.

"Marnie," I say. "I can't help noticing how wary you are of Tom getting aroused. It's like you think of it as some kind of demand on you."

"Well, isn't it? He needs to come, doesn't he?"

"Well, actually no. He's not fourteen anymore. It's not like he's going to burst from too much hydraulic pressure. And if he wants to have an orgasm, he knows how to give himself one."

"You mean while we're lying in bed together?" She's startled by the idea.

"Whatever you both feel comfortable with. It's not such a big deal."

This is a surprise to her. "I always thought it *was* a big deal," she says.

Tom giggles. Then Marnie hits him with her purse, and he laughs out loud.

The Talking Cure

I see Marnie and Tom in the office a week later.

"I did what you recommended," Marnie says. "I spent some time alone just tuning in to my breath and my body. It was really nice—except this sadness of mine kept creeping in. When that happened, I just tried to let it be—like you said."

Then she tells me what happened when they tried no-touch in bed:

"I remember you said we could talk, and all of a sudden *all* I wanted to do was talk. About how tired I was. And how weird it is to always feel so discouraged when I have two healthy, beautiful children.

"Then I started to cry, and I couldn't stop. It felt good to cry like that. I know I wasn't supposed to have Tom touch me, but I just needed him to hold me, and he did."

She sighs. "I guess that was cheating, but it felt like such a relief."

"Then what happened?"

"I think we both fell asleep."

"Did you figure out what was upsetting you?"

"I don't think it was any one thing in particular. Just everything all together. Trying to juggle work and the kids. Feeling like I never have time to do anything really well anymore. Tom's mother driving me crazy. Ordinary stuff."

She turns to Tom. "By the way, I really appreciated your letting me vent about your mother."

"I just tried to think of it as foreplay," he says. "That helped."

She moves to hit him again with her purse, but he catches her just in time.

A few weeks go by, and Marnie and Tom continue to lie down together whenever they're able. Often Marnie finds she needs a few minutes to complain about all her frustrations, and sometimes to cry a little. She says this really helps, and she really looks forward now to Tom holding her afterward.

I'm thrilled that she finds his physical presence to be a positive experience. Her "talking cure" in bed with Tom is a bit unusual, but it seems to be helping.

As a Two-Step strategy (Chapter 6), Marnie's talking and crying and being held seems to be a nice step one. I wonder whether she might be ready for step two—which as you'll recall is when you start to introduce arousal.

Marnie seems to be wondering the same thing.

"Okay," she asks at their next appointment. "When are we going to get to some actual sex?"

"You feel ready?" I ask her.

"I think so," she says.

"So go for it. When Tom holds you, just let yourself feel aroused."

She laughs. "We're already doing a lot of that! When can we have *sex?*"

"Oh, you mean intercourse."

She nods, blushing.

"Whenever you want," I say. "But just one thing. Don't make it simply a matter of humping and pumping to try to get off. Try to hold on to that honest, alive feeling—even after he goes inside you."

Marnie turns to Tom. "You got that?" she asks him.

"Got it," he says.

Bedroom Talk

Many couples take a vow of silence in bed.
That's not usually such a great idea.

"One more thing," I tell them before they leave the office. "You might want to keep talking to each other during step two."

"About *what?*" Marnie asks warily.

"Whatever you need, and whatever you feel."

Tom is nodding his head, so I know he gets it. Marnie seems doubtful.

"It's an advanced technique," I tell her.

"Explain," she asks.

I turn to Tom.

"'Tom,'" I say, "'when you go inside me, I just want you to hold me so I can feel close to you for a moment.'"

"I like that," says Tom. "But it would be even nicer if Marnie said it."

Marnie giggles.

"Or how about, 'Tom, I'm really tired tonight, but I can tell you're excited. What do you think we should do?'"

"I can see how that might be useful," says Marnie.

Marnie and Tom experiment with this kind of verbal intimacy

in bed, and it ends up saving them a lot of misunderstandings. Here's an example, as they're getting ready for bed one night.

Let's listen in:

Tom: *Your body is turning me on.*

Marnie: *Oh, Tom, you know I can't right now.*

Tom: *Marnie, all I said was that your body was turning me on. It wasn't a demand.*

Marnie: *Okay, thanks for explaining! (She thinks for a moment.) You know, if you want to simmer with me for a few minutes, I'd be good with that.*

Tom: *If I simmer with you right now, I'm going to need an orgasm.*

Marnie: *Can you come by grinding up against me?*

Tom: *I think so. But only if you let me finger you at the same time.*

Marnie: *Okay, but wash your hands first. And make it quick. No trying to get me excited. This is just for your sake. I've got to get to sleep.*

Tom: *Thanks, babe.*

Marnie: *Hey, no problem.*

Tom: *I'm glad we can talk like this.*

Marnie: *Me too.*

As you can see, it's all in the details.

~~~

Marnie and Tom end up having a lot of fun with step two.

I tell them they also shouldn't forget step one. A lot of couples forget about step one, once they're feeling better.

Which is a shame, really. But what are you gonna do?

Afterword

I don't want to give you the impression that helping someone regain desire is always this easy. It's definitely not.

Not all men have as good a feel for nondemand arousal as Tom. In fact, most men need a lot of coaching about this. And not all women who are as depressed as Marnie will get better just from couple's therapy alone.

But most couples in this situation can benefit from recognizing their sex-knots, talking honestly about their emotions, and possibly doing some mindfulness practice that helps them focus on what they're actually feeling.

You might say every couple has a "sexual bank account" together. Whenever you have good sex or an intimate conversation about real feelings, it's as if you're making a deposit in your account.

Keep putting money in that account, and it can pay you a handsome return someday when you need it. We'll talk about that much more in Part III.

But first I need to talk with you about a more difficult problem: What to do when it's the *man* who doesn't want sex.

That's not supposed to happen, right?

Unfortunately, it does. More and more these days.

The fact that it's not supposed to happen can make it a much more worrisome experience.

Why Men Go Missing in Bed

Most straight men tend to hear any female unhappiness as criticism.

This leads to all sorts of mischief for heterosexual couples.

"Many men are actually highly sensitive to evidence that their partners are unhappy or unsatisfied, feeling that the satisfaction of women, like that of their mothers, is their responsibility and yet almost impossible to achieve."
—MICHAEL BADER, *MALE SEXUALITY*

The first thing David tells me when he sits down in my office is that he's only here because his wife, Gwen, insisted on it.

"She's going to leave me," he says, "unless I start initiating sex."

David is a handsome man with a good-natured smile. Given the situation, he looks surprisingly relaxed.

David tells me his wife found my name online.

"Is she going to join us?" I ask.

"No. She insisted I see you alone."

"Why?"

"She says she's tired of trying to fix me."

Hmm. That doesn't sound good.

It's also a sign of the times. A few generations ago, men would send their wives to doctors to be "fixed"—for "frigidity," "hysteria," or whatever.

Now the shoe's definitely on the other foot. Now it's usually women who send their husbands to be fixed. Some days I get so many calls from women whose male partners have gone missing in bed that it feels like they must all be sharing notes.

Over the last few years I've seen so many couples like this that by now I'm practically a specialist in it. Usually the trouble is more emotional than sexual—as we'll see.

"Are you still physically attracted to her?" I ask him.

David says he is, and that when they have sex he still gets turned on.

"So what happens when you try to initiate sex?"

"That's the problem," he says. "It's like there's this invisible force field that stops me."

"Any idea what that's about?"

"Not really. All day long at work, I'll be thinking about how when I get home I'm going to start something up with her. But the closer I get to home, the less I feel like it."

"Why? What happens?"

"I don't know. She's usually complaining about one thing or another. She works hard. But I work hard too, and after a long day I really don't feel like listening to her complain."

He shifts in the chair. "Most of the time, I end up just shutting her out."

"I assume she doesn't like that very much."

"Yeah, she hates it. She never stops talking about how I never pay her any attention."

He stops for a moment and looks around the room.

"To tell you the truth, I don't think she likes me very much anymore."

What Men Really Want

It's commonly assumed that men automatically want sex. And in fact most men do respond automatically to attractive body parts.

Young or old, gay or straight, men tend to be pretty simple that way.

But male sexuality is only so automatic if we're talking about *looking*. In a real situation with a partner, a man ordinarily needs more. That's where it can get complicated.

You know how most women need to feel desired?

Most straight men need to feel *welcomed*.

There's a certain smile a woman wears when she's really pleased—a big, welcoming smile of pleasure that says, "Hey, I'm so glad you showed up! Come on in!"

That big, welcoming smile means it's okay to proceed, and you don't have to worry about *vagina dentata* or any other such hazards. That smile has been on the face of every woman in *Playboy* since forever—which of course is no accident.

Gay relationships can be somewhat different. But in male-female intimacy, the woman's body is where sex "happens." He's only a visitor there. He needs to know it's safe to enter.

When is a man's desire most likely to be "automatic," in the classical way that male libido is usually depicted?

In a new relationship, of course.

When a couple is just getting started, everyone is in a good mood most of the time. She smiles at him a lot, and the resultant boost to his sense of self gives him a perpetual green light to go ahead.

The trouble often starts when a man first sees his partner disappointed or unhappy. Especially if he's the *source* of her disappointment or unhappiness.

When that happens, his desire can become a lot less automatic.

Men get used to being the object of women's approval or disapproval when they are boys. Mothers criticize. So do wives. The echoes of a man's childhood experiences in this regard are often very much present when he lets an adult woman into his life.

David leans back in my office chair and looks up at the ceiling.

"Tell me," I ask him. "Were you and Gwen happy at the beginning, when you first started out together?"

"Yeah, it was great," he says. "We worked hard and played hard, and the sex was awesome."

"Do you remember when that changed?"

"I think it was when we moved in together. All of a sudden it was like everything I did was wrong. It's been that way ever since."

The Straight Man's Dilemma

According to the conventional script, a man is supposed to act like a leader. If he feels criticized or unaccepted, he can't just pout or cry or act needy. Instead, he'll usually just try to adopt as confident a pose as he can, and hope his hurt feelings will pass.

This tends not to work so well, of course, since his sexual self doesn't have the necessary coping skills to pull it off.

Eventually, out of desperation, a man who feels criticized or unaccepted will usually just withdraw. That's something few women appreciate, or even understand.

He feels criticized, so he withdraws.

This makes her angry, and even more critical of him.

He withdraws further—and so on, and so on.

When he withdraws emotionally, he'll often withdraw sexually too.

She'll of course usually interpret that to mean he doesn't desire her anymore. Which as you know is very bad.

A woman who no longer feels desired will almost never show a man that special welcoming smile of hers. Which of course he'll take to mean that it's no longer safe to approach her.

Which of course is totally nuts, since the only reason she never smiles anymore is because he hasn't touched her in a month—but that's the way these things tend to go.

Ultimately even the most self-assured woman may lose her temper, question whether he's gay or having an affair, and demand to know what's going on—leading to what must surely be the mother of all male-female sex-knots:

He has no desire for her.

She freaks out and gets upset with him.

Now he *really* has no desire for her.

By the time it's gotten to this point, he's usually lost all confidence in his ability to make her happy. He may try to make the best of the situation, by being good to her in other ways. Or he may regress to silly, childish behavior—like telling stupid jokes, or pulling pranks.

He may just try to act like everything's okay. But he and she both know these are all just poses—and that underneath he's in despair because his confidence is gone.

Most women will tell you that male confidence is a key ingredient for male sexiness. A man losing his confidence is like a woman losing faith in her power to attract. It's a very bad thing.

Can This Marriage Be Saved?

Let's get back to David.

"What would you most like to accomplish in here?" I ask.

David leans back again in the chair. "You know, this really wasn't my idea. But I'd like it if she didn't criticize me so much."

"Good," I say—a little too eagerly, I'm sure, but relieved to have found someplace practical to start. "Let's do it."

He looks surprised. "Do *what?*"

"Let's get her not to criticize you so much."

He gives me a wry look. "And just how are *we* going to do *that?*"

"Easy. We're going to cure her of her loneliness," I say.

"Who said she was lonely?"

"When a women criticizes a man as much as Gwen has been criticizing you," I tell him, "it almost always means she's lonely. Women only get shrill like that because they think no one's listening. Stop running away, and let's see what happens."

David agrees to try not running away from Gwen. And to turn off his smartphone when they talk—something she's been trying to get him to do for years. When he does, he's surprised to find her quite interested in talking about all sorts of other things besides his flaws.

But sex is another matter. David is still unable—or unwilling (it's often hard to tell)—to initiate anything in bed. They still have sex once in a while, but it's always Gwen initiating.

Weeks go by, and he and I discuss the subject every which way. But nothing changes.

Finally, feeling stuck, I get David's permission to call Gwen on the phone.

"I'm sorry," she says. "But I don't have the energy to go through this anymore. Either he has to show me some desire, or I'm done."

I end up offering her a deal:

Meet with me once, and I'll never bother you again.

She reluctantly agrees.

Gwen's Side of the Story

A week later, Gwen takes off her coat and sits down in my office. She's an elegant woman who looks like she's been working too hard. We end up talking for an hour and a half, and she tells me the story of their relationship from the beginning.

Gwen says that when she first met David, she'd never have guessed things would end up this way. She never met a man who made her feel so *special.*

David had boundless energy and was always full of creative ideas for things to do. He wasn't the best lover Gwen had ever known, but he was certainly the most warmhearted and enthusiastic—and that largely made up for it.

When he proposed to her, it was at a big event he'd staged—with all their friends looking on. She'd said yes without a moment's hesitation. But after they moved in together, she noticed something was off.

"Sometimes David and I would be talking," she says. "He'd ask me a question, and then ten minutes later he'd ask me the same question again. He just wasn't *there*. It was like now that he had me, he could just forget about me and move on to the next challenge.

"And then all of a sudden he stopped wanting sex. I figured maybe he was having an affair, so I looked through all his devices. Nothing. A little porn here and there, but that's it. He's a good soul, and I know he really loves me. But I can't go on feeling ignored like this."

She thinks for a moment. "He's also extremely disorganized," she adds. "I'm not the neatest person in the world, but it's stressful always having to pick up after him."

"What do you think the problem is?" I ask her.

"I wondered if he might have ADHD," she says. "But he concentrates just fine at work when there's a big business deal on the table."

"That's actually typical for people with ADHD," I say. "It's not really 'attention *deficit*' at all. It's just trouble focusing on things that aren't immediately exciting."

Gwen looks down, trying not to cry. "I guess I can deal with the fact that he doesn't find me that exciting anymore. But it still kind of hurts."

Chipmunk Love

Among the couples I see, it's very common for one partner's ADHD to be at the root of a lot of mischief—both in their family of origin and later when they get married.

Here's a famous example. See if you can identify who in the following script has ADHD:

"Simon?"
"Yes, Dave."
"Theodore?"
"Yes, Dave."
"Alvin? . . . Alvin?! . . . ALVIIIN!!!!!"

Yes, of course it's Alvin—who was no doubt absorbed in something else and didn't notice his name being called.

Whoever wrote those lines lived through something painful—as a kid, as a parent, or both—and managed to transform it into comedy.

In its original human form it was definitely not funny.

The Alvins of the world get yelled at a lot. A parent may do their best to be kind, but when everyone else is hurrying to get out the door for an important family event—all except little Alvin, who has his shoes off in front of the TV, completely unaware of the time or of what's going on around him—you're going to hear some yelling.

Many ADHD boys, like Alvin, are naturally resilient in the face of all the criticism they receive. When they grow up, that resilience can make them outstanding battlefield generals, trauma surgeons, and captains of industry. But that doesn't mean they're not traumatized.

The other side of the encounter can be just as traumatic. A wife can feel indescribably lonely when her grown-up Alvin is so absorbed with his iPad that he doesn't even hear her calling his name. Over the course of many years, she may end up saying things to him that she never imagined would ever come out of her mouth.

Sometimes they're the same things that Alvin's mother used to say. So it will all feel vaguely familiar to him. Often he'll react the same way he did as a boy—by shutting her out.

All Kinds of Male Minds

A good sex therapist will learn as much as they can about a man's specific mental assets and vulnerabilities. Some men have short attention spans and get easily bored in bed. Some use sex to self-medicate anxiety and need to have it all the time. Some get so distracted by other things that they forget about sex entirely.

Some have poor memories and keep doing the same thing over and over, even after their partner has told them she hates it. Some don't understand emotions at all. And some have various other quirks that aren't so easily categorized but can make them equally frustrating as partners.

These days we therapists often refer to all these kinds of men as "atypical."

Many women are atypical as well. But for some reason a woman's atypicality doesn't seem to come up as often as an issue in sex therapy—at least not in heterosexual couples.

A man's neuropsychological vulnerabilities, though, are frequently an issue in treatment. It's as if he's in double jeopardy—both from being atypical, and from being a man.

"It's not just about sex," says Gwen. "Sometimes I just want to know he's thinking about me. It would mean a lot if he would just wipe the kitchen counter once in a while. But he never even notices it's dirty."

"I wonder why you chose David in the first place," I ask. "I'm sure you had lots of other opportunities."

"Maybe I wanted adventure," she says, looking very unhappy. "Maybe I'm just not cut out for adventure. Right now, I just need someone to notice that the kitchen counter needs cleaning. Maybe I'm shallow that way."

She looks at her watch and tells me she has to go. She gets up to put on her coat.

"Can you tell me why he doesn't want to have sex with me anymore?" she asks.

"Maybe because he feels you criticize him all the time," I say.

"I know. I try hard not too. But I'm so disappointed. I guess I don't hide that very well."

She thinks for a moment. "I thought men automatically want sex."

"Yeah, everybody thinks that. The truth is, we're just like women. We need to feel appreciated."

She gives me a sad smile, shakes my hand, and leaves—closing the door carefully behind her.

David Again

The next time I see David, we spend some time with my adult ADHD checklist.

David has a few hyperactive symptoms, but it's his inattentive symptoms that really clinch the diagnosis. Trouble finishing things, chronic lateness, trouble staying organized. A tendency to lose his keys, to tune out during conversations, and to make careless mistakes when he's bored. He tells me the only way he got through college was by shutting himself up in the library basement so he wouldn't get distracted.

I'm always amazed that people like David can get to adulthood without anyone suspecting they might have ADHD. Even today most people, including most therapists, miss the diagnosis completely—especially with someone like David who's very smart and has what Gina Pera, the author of *Is It You, Me, or Adult A.D.D.?* calls "stealth ADD"*—mostly inattentive, without much hyperactivity.

Stealth ADHD tends to fly under most people's radar screens.

---

* "ADD" and "ADHD" mean the same thing. ADHD is the more up-to-date term. It's possible to have ADHD with or without hyperactivity.

I end up trying David on several different ADHD medications before we find one he likes. After several months, David marvels at how he could ever have managed without it.

I'm eager to see what will happen between Gwen and David, now that he's gotten some help for his ADHD. But I know from experience that these things are always complicated, so I'm not expecting any miracles.

You can't necessarily generalize from David and Gwen's story to all couples. Obviously not every man in David's situation has ADHD. And not every person with ADHD has relationship problems.

But it's very common for couples in treatment to have at least one partner with this condition. Often they've been in therapy for years without their therapist ever considering the possibility. So I felt I had to mention it.

12

Standing Your Ground

Your partner should accept you for who you are.
If they don't, then you may need to insist on it.

"Sometimes . . . a man requires help in being actively asser-
tive. He needs to do as he pleases with his partner, or to tell her
what to do. The requests he may learn to make are occasionally
as simple as, 'Please move your elbow; it's in my ribs.'"
—AVODAH OFFIT, NIGHT THOUGHTS

Several months have now passed, and I don't know whether it's
mostly the medicine or our work together, but there's been a nice
change in David. He carries himself with more dignity. He seems
more thoughtful. More fully grown-up.

David says he never realized how bad he'd always felt about himself, and how much he'd hidden himself from Gwen. Now he's
eager to make up for lost time with her. He's even started initiating sex again.

But David is worried about Gwen. He says lately she just seems
to be going through the motions. A couple of times he's found her
crying in bed at night when she thought he was asleep, and both
times he asked her what it was and she just shook her head and said
nothing.

Now it's Gwen who seems to have gone missing.

This happens sometimes in couples. Someone changes in an important way, and their partner responds by getting depressed.

Sometimes it's because there's been too much change.

Sometimes it's that there hasn't been enough.

Often it's both—which can be terribly confusing.

One day David tells me that Gwen has asked to come in to see me with him. I say okay, and the following week they're in my waiting room together.

It's an anxious moment. I have no idea what I'm going to hear—but from what David tells me about the way Gwen's been acting lately, I'm pretty sure it's not going to be good.

I go out to the waiting room and invite them in.

Now David and Gwen are sitting side by side on my couch, both staring ahead.

"Where should we start?" I ask.

Gwen answers first. "I want to thank you for helping David," she says. "He's so much happier—more like the man I fell in love with."

She pauses, and her eyes look away, wet. "But I don't know how to do this anymore."

He gives her a questioning look.

"It's always like a project for him, to get me back. Once I open up to him again, he goes away."

She turns to face him on the sofa and takes hold of his hand. "David, how do I know a year from now you won't go back to disappearing again?"

"I need you to trust me," he says.

She swallows. "Actually, that's just one thing."

"Tell me the others," he says.

"A lot of times you still don't *notice* me. I know you love me, but I don't *feel* it."

"I do notice you."

"You notice me more in bed—which I definitely appreciate. But the rest of the time I still only get your attention for a few seconds, then I'm left hanging."

"You have my attention right now."

"That's just because we're in Dr. Snyder's office. It's like when I get angry that you've left your stuff everywhere. You'll make an effort for a day or two, but it doesn't last. I'm tired of feeling like your mother."

She looks down at her lap and smooths out her dress.

"Lately I keep having this memory," she says. "I'm eleven years old, and it's my first night back in my own bed after summer camp. I get into bed and I feel the bedsheets—cool against my skin—and I know my mother made the bed all straight and nice so it would feel good when I got home.

"I need to be loved like that," she says. "Not just in the big picture, but in all the little details. David just isn't a details kind of guy—even on medication."

Standing Your Ground

So where do we go from here?

I'm feeling unexpectedly hopeful. Gwen is speaking plainly, and David isn't backing down or apologizing. They're both staying reasonably calm. One might say they're both "standing their ground." That tends to be a good sign.

I'm also getting an idea about why they married each other in the first place. Should I try to explain it to them? Better to get more information first.

"Gwen," I say, "can I ask you more about this memory—the one where you come home from summer camp?"

She looks surprised at my bringing it up again, but happy that I was paying attention.

"It sounds like a lonely memory," I tell her.

"What do you mean?" she says.

"There aren't any *people* in it."

She smiles. "I don't remember it feeling lonely. I liked being alone. It was relaxing."

"Can you tell me about your mother?"

"She's very detail-oriented. Just like me. She can also be kind of critical sometimes."

"People who are good with details are *usually* kind of critical."

"Why *is* that?"

"I don't know. Maybe because they notice things that other people don't notice, and it drives them crazy. Was your mother happy?"

"As happy as a perfectionist like her could be. There was always something she wasn't satisfied with. That could be hard sometimes."

"She criticized you?"

"She criticized everyone. I think I got that from her. She's always been better with linens than with people."

"I think in this memory of yours, your mother's bedsheets might stand in for her full physical self. It's a compromise: You get to enjoy her attention without having to endure her actual presence. Kind of brilliant."

Gwen listens intently, trying to put this all together.

"I think one reason you married David is because you knew he'd never criticize you. You can tolerate solitude okay, but criticism is the one thing you can't stand."

"How could I have known David wouldn't criticize me?" she asks, intrigued.

"Because he never looks closely enough to notice your flaws. He's like Alvin from *Alvin and the Chipmunks*. He's basically just a happy guy who wants to have fun."

We both turn to David. He gives us a wide grin and two thumbs-up.

"*I'd* like to be able to have fun like that," says Gwen.

"Some people are naturally better at it than others," I say.

David crosses his eyes and sticks out his tongue sideways like a big letter Q. Gwen laughs.

"Do you think there's any hope for us?" she asks, sighing.

"Actually, I have lots of hope. You're each self-sufficient, in your own way. You had to be, or you'd both have been criticized to death growing up. That's a great strength you both have."

"Why are we having all these problems?"

"Because neither of you has much confidence that you can advocate for your own needs in the presence of someone else. I think that's why you married each other. To learn to do that."

"So you don't think we made a mistake getting married?"

"Right now you're suffering together honestly. That can be the royal road to happiness for a couple, if you learn to do it right."

She gives me a cockeyed look. "You think suffering is a good thing?"

"Only if you do it right," I say.

The Dance of Intimacy

We cannot make another person change his or her steps to an old dance, but if we change our steps, the dance no longer can continue in the same predictable pattern.

—HARRIET LERNER, THE DANCE OF ANGER

In the late 1950s, around the same time Masters and Johnson started observing people having sex in the lab, psychiatrist Murray Bowen spent five years at the National Institute of Mental Health observing the families of hospitalized mental patients.

Bowen's methods were extremely curious, to say the least. A patient would be admitted to the hospital along with his or her *entire immediate family*—and the whole family would live there for months, having their every interaction monitored by the staff.

After years of watching families up close, Bowen felt he finally understood how families worked. His findings, first published in

1966, launched a revolution in how the mental health profession thinks about people and relationships.

Bowen taught that in most families people just react to each other without thinking much, and as a consequence they just keep doing the same painful things over and over again. He called these families "poorly differentiated." They tend to get wrapped up in each other's emotions, and as a result everyone is highly anxious most of the time.

In *well-differentiated* families, things are different. They have a stronger sense of themselves as individuals. They don't just react to each other's emotions. As a result, they tend to be a lot less anxious.

Being well-differentiated doesn't mean keeping your distance. In fact, it's the opposite. If you know how to stay emotionally balanced in the presence of someone you care about, you'll be more likely to stay emotionally engaged.

Well-differentiated people tend to have an easier time tolerating conflict and disagreement in relationships. Whereas poorly differentiated people tend to get so flooded with emotion that they need to run away. Or they suppress important parts of themselves in order to keep the peace.

David could stay emotionally engaged with Gwen as long as she was happy with him. But the minute she expressed disappointment he crumbled and had to run away.

Now David is acting differently. He's no longer quite so reactive to Gwen's disappointment. He's become better differentiated. As a result he's much less anxious—and a lot more courageous.

You'd think David's newfound ability to stand his ground with Gwen would make her happy. But so far her reaction has been mostly negative.

I think David's therapy with me has helped him differentiate. But Gwen hasn't had that opportunity yet. Maybe if Gwen could differentiate too, she might be able to stand her ground better.

In 1985 Harriet Lerner wrote *The Dance of Anger*, based partly on Bowen's principles. Now almost thirty years later, *The Dance of*

Anger is still an excellent guide to taking responsibility for your own emotional well-being in a relationship. Her cautious, methodical approach is one that millions of readers have found helpful.

Lerner writes about seeking a balance between the "I" and the "we" in a marriage. That's obviously important for sex as well. But sex was never Lerner's primary focus.

It wasn't until 1991, when David Schnarch published his major theoretical work, *Constructing the Sexual Crucible*, that we sex therapists finally had a theory of sex based on Bowen's principles.

Schnarch taught that most couples originally bond together based on what he called "other-validated intimacy." They lean on each other for approval.

But no relationship can sustain itself forever that way. Sooner or later, the well of mutual approval runs dry and each of you needs to stand your own ground.

Marriage, according to Schnarch, gives you an opportunity to learn "self-validated intimacy."

You take responsibility for your own emotions, rather than just leaning on your partner for approval.

The kind of emotional self-control we're talking about here isn't as important at the start of a relationship. But as a relationship progresses, you have to learn to stand your ground or the sex may start to wane.

Back to the Bedroom

Marriage asks, "Are you willing to stand up now, or do things have to get worse?"
—DAVID SCHNARCH, *INTIMACY AND DESIRE*

I decide it's time to ask David and Gwen about sex.

David is the first to speak. "To tell you the truth," he says, "I'm a little frustrated."

Gwen looks surprised.

"You still hurry me through foreplay," he says. "Like you want to get it over with."

She thinks for a moment. "Maybe I'm worried you'll suddenly stop paying attention," she whispers sadly. "That's been known to happen."

"That was before," he says, "when I felt so hopeless about being able to make you happy."

"And now?"

"Your happiness is up to you. All I can do is enjoy you, if you'll let me."

Gwen turns to me.

"I honestly don't know," she says. "He's saying all these sweet things, and I can see he's changed. But it still doesn't feel safe."

"What are you going to do?" I ask.

"I don't know," she says. "It's tearing me apart."

"I have an idea," I say. "Start small. Start with foreplay."

Gwen gives me a puzzled look.

"David says he just wants to enjoy your body. But that's scary. You don't know if it's safe to let yourself enjoy his attention. Maybe he'll leave you frustrated again."

"What do you suggest?" she asks.

"Feel scared, I guess. Just stay with it. See what happens."

"I don't like feeling scared."

"No one does," I tell her. "But feelings come and go. I'd be interested in what you might feel next, after the scared feeling passes."

"There's no guarantee I won't get disappointed again."

"Tell David you can't offer him any guarantees either."

She looks at David and takes his hand.

"Okay," she says. "I'm in."

The Courage to Feel

Being deeply loved by someone gives you strength.
Loving someone deeply gives you courage.
—LAO TZU

Months later, Gwen and I talk about the change that happened that day in my office when they both stood their ground.

"I liked that he didn't back down," she says. "And that he told me he really wanted me. Before then, I felt he was just being a dutiful boy, and the minute I let down my guard he'd go running off again."

Gwen gets quiet for a moment. "You know, for years I've been thinking about leaving him."

"What made you stay?"

"Maybe I knew I'd find fault with the next one too. David is a good man. I just couldn't manage to feel anything for him anymore."

"Can you feel anything for him now?" I ask.

"Sometimes I do, and sometimes I don't. I'm learning not to give myself such a hard time about that. But it's still scary when it doesn't happen."

Gwen thinks some more. "It helped that you said it was okay to suffer."

"Yeah, suffering's all right—as long as you stand your ground."

"I didn't understand that at all. But then we did it in your office, and it made sense."

"How did it go with the foreplay?" I ask.

"Very enlightening. It helped just to concentrate on my own feelings. I realized I'd been so worried he was going to lose focus, that I completely lost my own focus."

Gwen looks uncertain for a moment, as if taking stock of the fact that she's about to tell me something more intimate.

"I also realized I'd never really enjoyed intercourse. It was just the price you paid for getting a man."

She blushes. "Sometimes lately I just tell him to hold still, while I grind against *him*. That works much better."

"Is he okay with it?"

"At this point he's okay with anything that makes me happy."

"Does he still get distracted sometimes?" I ask.

"Sometimes," she says. "But I just try to stay with my own arousal. A lot of times that brings him back. In the past I used to go chasing after him. That never worked."

Gwen gives me a proud look. "I think I'm learning that if you feel disappointed it doesn't have to be a catastrophe. It's just a feeling."

"A lot of people never learn that," I say.

"I know," she says. "I almost missed the opportunity myself."

Beyond the Conventional Script

Remember the "conventional script" from Chapter 7? He leads, she follows. He's in control, but she's the main object of attention.

The more you differentiate in a relationship, the less you need to be bound by conventional gender expectations. A woman can take charge, for instance. A man can give up control. And intercourse doesn't always have to be the main thing on the menu.

But the conventional script is very powerful. You have to have a certain tolerance for anxiety if you want to start breaking the rules.

For gays and lesbians and most other members of sexual minorities, it's impossible to be who you are *without* breaking the rules. Sometimes you have to tolerate anxiety just to *exist*.

In previous generations, it was common for gay men and lesbians to spend their whole lives in the closet. But that just traded one form of anxiety for another.

In the last couple of decades in many parts of the West, it's become more acceptable for a member of a sexual minority to come out as to who they really are. But it can take years to build up the courage to do so.

Only in the past few years has it been possible for significant numbers of gay and lesbian young people to reach adolescence without ever having had to hide their sexual identity. That's a monumental change.

It's a serious act of differentiation though to come out at any age as gay, lesbian, bisexual, transgender, gender-nonconforming, or just very kinky.

And even after you've done so, you'll probably still need to differentiate further in order to feel fully yourself in a long-term relationship.

That's true no matter who you are.

Sarina Finds a New Partner

We first met Sarina in Chapter 2 when she came out to herself about being lesbian. One day several years later I get a call from Sarina saying she wants help with her new live-in partner Jo.

Like many lesbian couples, Sarina and Jo tend to take turns during lovemaking. Sex usually starts with Sarina bringing Jo to climax. But when it's Sarina's turn to receive pleasure from Jo, Sarina often can't relax enough to enjoy it. Jo seems too tentative—too worried about doing it right. Sarina wants Jo to take charge and be more aggressive.

Jo wants acceptance. "I just don't think I'm much of a take-charge person in bed," she says.

"Yeah, but I need that," says Sarina.

"You may need it," says Jo. "But that doesn't make it my responsibility to give it to you."

Somehow Jo's decision to stand her ground like this gives the relationship a spark of energy. They decide to get creative. Maybe they should switch and have Jo give *Sarina* the first orgasm.

That works much better. When Jo isn't postorgasmic, it's easier for her to express desire in a way that Sarina can feel.

One day when they're about to make dinner, Jo kisses Sarina passionately and tells her to lie down and close her eyes. This excites Sarina very much, and she's much more responsive when Jo brings her to orgasm.

"Let's do that again," says Sarina.

"I don't know," says Jo. "I'm not sure that's really *me*."

"I understand," says Sarina.

Sarina's understanding makes Jo feel more relaxed and accepted, and after a while the erotic climate in the relationship improves to where it no longer really matters who has the first orgasm.

In retrospect, Sarina and Jo decide the issue was never really much about sex at all. It was about each of them feeling accepted for who they are.

Adam

Adam remembers being ten years old and realizing he's nothing like his father. His father seems naturally comfortable with his own body, in a way that Adam can only envy.

Adam's friends remind him of his father. They like rough-and-tumble sports, horsing around, teasing each other—things Adam doesn't like at all. From the age of ten, Adam is sure there's something wrong with him, and prays every night to be fixed.

Adam never develops an interest in girls. He mostly just envies girls and wishes he could be one. He likes their easy sensuality, their deep conversations with each other, and the fact that they don't have to pretend to enjoy sports.

It takes Adam a long time to fall in love. When he does, at twenty-five, it's with a man. In retrospect, Adam realizes this has been coming for a long time. He just hadn't been ready to face it.

By the time Adam comes to see me at fifty, he's a top entertainment lawyer who splits his time between New York and Los Angeles. He and Seth have been together for two years. Seth is a good decade younger than Adam and wants to get married. Adam isn't sure.

"He's too feminine," Adam says. "I fantasize about being with a man who doesn't look so gay."

I listen to Adam's account of his growing up, and I search the man in front of me for any trace of the sensitive boy he says he used to be.

"What happened to that boy?" I ask.

"It was a different world back then. I envy gay boys growing up today. They don't have to pretend to be someone they're not."

"Maybe you're envious of Seth. By the time he was born, the world was more open to difference. He doesn't have to playact someone else's idea of masculinity."

"It doesn't feel like envy. It feels like disgust."

I think for a moment, wondering how to get behind Adam's armor of contempt.

"Look," I say. "I grew up in the same world you did. I know the whole male drill: sports, fistfights, stupid pranks. I hated it too."

"Are you gay?"

"No. But I know a little bit about growing up thinking there's something wrong with you."

Adam studies me carefully. Then he looks away and is quiet for a long time.

"Any advice?"

"Next time you feel disappointed with Seth, just notice the feeling. Breathe into it. Be aware you're pushing him away because of something in yourself you haven't reconciled with."

"That sounds hard."

"It gets easier, the more you practice."

The world is ambivalent about femininity. It idealizes it, but it also hates it. It can be cute if a girl is a tomboy and wants to wear pants, but it's not so cute if a boy wants to wear a dress.

Not all gay men have feminine qualities—and many straight men do. Straight or gay, though, a man who expresses too much of his feminine side can run the risk of turning off his partner.

I've noticed that older gay men like Adam are more likely to be concerned. Younger gay men, raised in a more permissive era, tend to be more relaxed about the whole thing.

The yearnings of the erotic mind very often concern something in ourselves that feels missing. It's tempting to try to get your partner to complete you. But it's usually better to stay with your own sense of incompleteness until you can calm down about it.

That's part of standing your ground too.

PART III

Sex for Life

In Part I we discussed the nature of the sexual self.

In Part II we talked about sex and gender.

In Part III we're going to put these fragments together and look at becoming a lifelong committed couple—from starting out as partners in the first place, through the expectable crises of midlife, and beyond.

My focus will be on sexually exclusive long-term relationships. That's not the only option these days, but for a whole host of reasons most people today still want to be monogamous.

If you've absorbed the lessons in this book, you already know a lot about how to have good sex with someone you love. But you can have lots of good sex together and still after many years find yourself without any desire for your partner. Desire is a frequent casualty of domestic life.

There are lots of books on what to do about this—how to keep desire alive, or bring it back once it's gone. This is not one of those books.

In the chapters that follow, I'm going to show you a different approach to thinking about eros in long-term relationships.

The approach I'm going to recommend doesn't rely on desire at all. Instead, it involves turning inward to connect with your deepest sources of inspiration.

That's better than just trying to stimulate desire. It's also a much better way to stay connected for a lifetime—as I'll show you.

Interested?

Good.

Let's get started.

13

Eros and Faith

You could define faith a hundred different ways. I like to think of it as a kind of inner coherence that allows you to keep your balance in a relationship.

That doesn't mean you'll be happy all the time. It just means that when you're miserable, you'll still be able to stand your ground—and to trust that the eventual outcome will be okay.

"For myself I remember the kindness of your youth, the love of your bridal days; how you followed me into the wilderness, into an unsown land."
—JEREMIAH 2:2

Emily

Years later, when we've gotten to know each other better, Emily will tell me that her strongest memories from childhood are of when she'd lose her temper and her mother would tell her that she was too sensitive.

That always made Emily feel bad about herself—which obviously didn't do much to improve her mood. Things tended to get worse between them from that point on.

Emily couldn't help being sensitive. She seemed to have been born that way. Her mother said she'd always been a difficult child—hard to soothe and easy to upset.

Emily would try to act more composed—but then one of her brothers would say the wrong thing to her over dinner, and Emily wouldn't be able to stop crying and would have to go to her room.

Later that night, Emily's mother—by this point weary of what she felt were Emily's continual dramatics—would tell her she really needed to stop being so sensitive, or no one would ever be able to make her happy.

～～

Somehow this prediction of her mother's seemed to come true in Emily's marriage to Jay. They'd met when they were graduate students together, keeping each other company late nights in the lab. They'd bonded over a shared love of science and the fact that they were both confirmed insomniacs.

Jay was smart, handsome, emotionally stable, and Emily's parents liked him a lot—though Emily had to admit this made her both happy and uncomfortable at the same time.

Jay proposed to Emily after they'd been living together for several months. She took a while to consider his proposal, then finally said yes—which at first felt like a huge relief.

But after they were engaged, Emily couldn't help noticing that sex with Jay had started to leave her cold. The experience didn't touch her at all.

Emily figured it was probably just anxiety. She knew from experience that anxiety could be very good at making you feel nothing. But still she couldn't help worrying that maybe there was something wrong with their sexual connection.

Was she making a mistake to get married? She started to notice things about Jay that she didn't like. Silly, trivial things—like how he sometimes told jokes at inappropriate times. The more she brooded about these things, the less she felt like having sex with him.

Finally he asked her what was wrong and she burst into tears. "I just don't feel anything anymore when we have sex," she said.

It was probably the wrong thing to say, but that's what came out.

Jay tried to be understanding. He agreed it was probably just anxiety and told her everything would be okay. But the experience made him more tentative. And that ended up making her even more worried.

By now the invitations had been sent out, and gifts had started arriving. But every package on their doorstep just made her more anxious. All she could think of was how she'd probably have to return them all.

They got through the wedding okay, but on their honeymoon Emily still didn't feel anything when they had sex—a fact that by then she'd learned to keep to herself. She found herself faking orgasms, which felt horrible. And faking arousal, which felt even worse.

Then Jay started to find fault with *her*. He'd criticize her work schedule, the fact that she didn't cook, even the movies she wanted to see. Emily knew she'd started it all by being critical of him, but by then the whole thing had spun out of control. Finally he asked her for a divorce.

Years later, looking back, Emily felt she knew exactly what had gone wrong. She'd been too young. She hadn't had enough confidence in herself. And she'd still had her mother's voice in her head saying if she didn't stop being so sensitive then no one would ever be able to make her happy.

Emily knew that in some way she'd made that prediction come true—as if she was trying to prove her mother right. Though why she'd want to prove her mother right was a mystery she still couldn't figure out.

Your Inner Voices

There's a place in your mind where everyone who's ever been important to you, living or dead, still lives on. That place doesn't really have a name. But if you're like most people, you probably spend a lot of time there.

The people who inhabit that place in your mind still speak to you in pretty much the same voices they used when you originally knew them. In the mental health field we call these voices your "introjects."

Everyone has lots of introjects. It's universal. Depending on the kind of mind you were born with, and what kind of experiences you had growing up, your introjects will be mostly friendly or mostly not.

With any luck, the people who raised you were reasonably gentle, patient, and had confidence in you—so your introjects will be mostly positive ones. But every parent has moments when they act unloving. And even the best parent can't prevent every misunderstanding or darkness of the soul.

As a result, even if you're very self-assured you no doubt have negative introjects as well—those voices that scold you, shame you, and make you feel the way you felt during the most miserable moments of childhood.

It's important to have lots of positive introjects, so you know you're worthy of being loved and desired. Positive introjects tend to run quietly in the background so you never know they're there. If you're a reasonably confident person, chances are you have lots of them you don't even know about.

Negative introjects tend to be much more noticeable. They're the voices that speak to you the way your parents and teachers used to speak when they weren't happy with you.

Negative introjects can be useful for making sure you don't get careless or overconfident. Like tough-love parents, they can keep you out of trouble. But when they get out of hand, they can easily lead to the negative obsessions we discussed in Chapter 4. Negative introjects are among the chief causes of misery in relationships.

One way of looking at faith is that it's what happens when the balance between your positive and negative introjects is tipped in favor of the good ones. Too many negative introjects can weaken your faith.

Many people's experiences in life haven't left them with enough faith. So it falls to marriage, therapy, or some other close relationship to help them develop it.

Faith is not the same as religious belief. Some religious individuals have tremendous faith, and a relationship with God or with a religious community can be a wonderful anchor for faith. But other people use religion to compensate for a lack of faith. And some people of exceptional faith have no religion at all.

Emily and Sam

When Emily meets Sam, she is thirty-two and has a promising research career at a major university here in New York. She rather likes being single—especially the freedom it gives her to spend evenings and weekends writing grant proposals instead of having to keep someone else company.

Emily has never been particularly boy-crazy or baby-crazy, and she figures if she never gets married again or has kids that will probably be okay. But sometimes when she can't write or think anymore she makes herself a cup of tea and checks out the men on OkCupid—half to distract herself, and half from a sense of wanting to keep her options open.

She's seen Sam's profile a few times—a nice-looking guy in swim trunks at the beach. He trades bonds for a living, which sounds kind of boring.

Sam notices Emily's profile too, and is intrigued—but he decides she's probably too intellectual for him and moves on.

Then one day Sam puts up a new picture of himself—a close-up in a suit and tie at a fancy party. Emily has always been a sucker for a man all dressed up. She takes the bait and messages him.

Flattered, he responds right away, and they meet that weekend. They intend only to have brunch—but it is such a gorgeous spring day that Sam suggests they rent a boat on the lake in Central Park, and Emily happily says yes.

By the next weekend, they are a couple.

~~~

Not all relationships start off so quickly. But for most couples there's at least one moment—a sudden explosion of energy, when a new world seems created out of nothing. The energy given off in that explosion, if tended properly, can fuel a relationship for a lifetime.

Perhaps that's why people don't fall in love that often. It can take years to store up the necessary emotional supplies—like a cactus waiting years before putting out one flower.

We hardly know the people we fall in love with. But a tremendous amount of information gets exchanged between two people in the first couple of hours after they meet.

Little things—the turn of a man's head, or the way he handles the oars in a boat—can contain an extraordinary amount of information for someone who's primed to notice.

Feeling Unreal

One day early in their relationship, Sam leaves a slightly playful message on Emily's voicemail, and she gets offended, thinking he's making fun of her. He apologizes and they resolve the misunderstanding. But the next time he kisses her, Emily feels as if she can't breathe right, and she has an uncomfortable sense of not being fully there.

He asks if she's okay, and she says she's just a little overwhelmed.

"I love you," he says.

Yes, she thinks. *So far you do. But you don't know how emotional I can be.*

A few days later, Emily starts to feel disconnected again during sex—just like when she was married. She has a sinking feeling that the whole disaster of her previous marriage is about to happen again.

One afternoon when Emily is reading in bed, Sam comes and lies down beside her and starts nuzzling her neck.

"Sometimes, when I'm feeling really happy with you," she tells him, "it totally scares me."

Sam stops nuzzling long enough to ask what she's scared about.

"I'm scared I'll screw everything up," she says. And she tells him the story of her first marriage, and how eventually she stopped feeling anything.

"Has that ever happened with me?" he asks. "I mean, where you didn't feel anything?"

"No," she lies. "But I'm worried it could."

"Well, if that happens, promise you'll let me know."

"What would we do about it?"

"I don't know," he says. "We'll think of something." He goes back to nuzzling her neck.

It isn't much of a conversation, but she likes that he didn't get upset. That makes her feel a little bit better. And the next time they make love, Emily doesn't feel quite so anesthetized. As time goes on, she feels more and more like herself again. Emily is pretty sure that just having the courage to say *something* to Sam in the moment was helpful—even though she didn't tell him everything.

Courage is a big part of faith. It takes courage to have faith, and faith in turn rewards you with courage. It's like a muscle. The more you use it, the stronger it gets.

Emily also can't help wondering whether it's different now because she's divorced. Her relationship with her ex-husband was so bound together with her ties to her family. Now she knows it's all up to her. That's lonelier, but better.

Emily still sometimes hears her mother's voice speaking to her—that harsh, worried voice she remembers from growing up. But now more and more, as Emily listens to the voice, she notices how much anxiety there's always been in it.

Emily was the only girl, so she'd naturally been the focus of all her mother's worries—but she hadn't understood them at all. Now lying next to Sam in the middle of the night, she considers her mother's words again: "No one will ever be able to make you happy."

That had been her mother's emotional universe, where a woman was supposed to find someone to make her happy.

Emily finds herself playing with her mother's words, turning them inside out.

"No," she thinks. "No one else will ever be able to make me happy. It's *my* job to take care of that."

Your negative introjects never entirely go away. They can still make themselves quite clearly heard in a moment of uncertainty or crisis. But if you're lucky, over time they get softened by more positive ones, as the voices of fear in your head get softened by calmer voices. Over time Sam's voice gets added to the choir of good introjects that sing Emily to sleep on those nights when she falls asleep most easily.

Emily hadn't anticipated that her relationship with Sam would challenge her faith in quite the way it did. But good relationships always challenge your faith. That's just how it is.

Emily's Talking Cure

Summer has turned to fall now, and Emily and Sam are still together. For several weeks, for some reason, Emily has found herself rather predictably crying when they have sex.

All of a sudden a yearning will start down near her clitoris and spread through her body—something like an orgasm, but made of pleasure and tears mixed together. Sometimes she'll be sobbing and coming all at the same time, and Sam will hold her as the waves of sobs rise and fall and then subside, leaving her body spent and her mind exhausted.

"Tear-gasms," she names them.

Sam gets so turned on by this that he comes right after her, just as her sobs are starting to subside. Both leaking from every port, they both laugh out loud sometimes at having gotten so carried away.

Emily never figures out exactly what the tears are all about. The feeling isn't exactly sadness. More like extreme vulnerability. Sometimes it's so disorienting it makes Emily want to go back to being single again.

~~~

One day after a particularly wet, tearful orgasm, Emily lies on top of Sam as he rocks her gently and kisses her shoulders.

"Do you remember what I told you about my first marriage?" she asks. "That after a while I couldn't feel anything—and you asked if that had ever happened with you?"

"I remember," he says.

"Actually, it did happen with you," she says into the pillow. "A few times early on. It always bothered me that I lied to you."

She pulls herself off him so she can see him more clearly, and they face each other, their heads on the pillows.

"I've been feeling so anxious and vulnerable lately," she tells him. "Do you ever feel that way?"

"No, not really."

"I feel that way all the time," she says. "The only thing that seems to help is when I tell you things that scare me."

She thinks for a moment. "Is there anything you want to tell *me*?" she asks.

"How about that you're the most emotional person I've ever met."

"*Too* emotional?"

"You really worry about that, don't you?"

"More than you could ever imagine."

Over the next few weeks, Emily tells Sam every shameful thing about herself she can recall. From the time she locked her younger brother in a closet, to the time she let herself get seduced by her thesis adviser. Everything.

She also makes it a point to tell him little things that she might ordinarily not tell him. Such as how one day in the kitchen she wishes he'd put his hands around her waist and tell her he loves her.

It seems strange to tell him this, rather than just wait to see if he'll do it. But at the same time it feels intimate and brave.

Emily likes this brave feeling. She still feels vulnerable a lot with Sam. And she still often cries during sex. But more and more when she cries, it's because she feels full of something good.

Red and Lavender

One day Emily finds herself in Midtown, looking for a birthday present for Sam. She finds a nice polo shirt for him, but she can't decide on the color.

Her favorite color is lavender. His is red. And it turns out the shirt is available in both of those colors. Should she get it in his favorite color, or hers?

Three days later Sam opens the box on his birthday, sees the lavender shirt in the wrapping paper, and smiles.

"Hey, is this for you, or for me?" he says.

"It's a little piece of me. Do you like it?"

"I love that it's a piece of you."

"You can exchange it for a red one."

"I wouldn't dream of it."

Did he really like it? Emily hopes so. She's glad she took the extra risk of giving him a piece of herself.

For some reason this reminds Emily of that O. Henry story from high school—"The Gift of the Magi"—where a young married woman who has no money on Christmas Eve sells her hair, the thing she loves best about herself, to buy her husband a strap for his prized watch. She doesn't know he's just sold his watch to buy her a set of combs for her wonderful hair.

Thinking it over, Emily realizes why she's always hated that story.

"If you love someone," she thinks, "don't give away what's best about you. Save it, so you can share it with the person you love. That's why they're with you in the first place."

Later Emily wonders if perhaps the story only came to mind because now she feels she has something good to share.

That's what faith does.

It makes you feel you have something good to share.

14

Becoming a Couple

Sooner or later, every relationship reaches a stage where you find yourself wondering why in the world you ever chose this person. That's normal. It's what you do once this happens that makes all the difference.

"The sexual is the most intimate world between two people. Into this milieu, where injured feelings buzz at the rafters like angry wasps, the sex therapist must move with gloved hands."
—AVODAH OFFIT, *THE SEXUAL SELF*

It's good to idealize your partner when you first fall in love. But idealization inevitably crumbles, leaving you sooner or later to realize that in certain ways large or small the two of you are fundamentally incompatible.

Once this happens, you have some options.

You can break up, of course. But let's assume you don't really want to.

You can change to accommodate your partner's needs—or try to get them to change to meet *your* needs. That doesn't usually work so well in the long term.

Instead it's usually much better to just tolerate feeling incompatible, if you can, and to just stand your ground.

It can be a rude shock at first to recognize how incompatible your needs are. That's your first test of faith. It's important that you be able to tolerate the suffering that goes with feeling incompatible, until the time comes when you eventually manage to build a new relationship that actually works for the two of you—where you're both able to get enough of what you need.

This new relationship, once you build it, will probably look different from what either of you originally had in mind. It also probably won't look exactly like the relationships you're familiar with from your own family.

But it will be yours. And you'll have finally become a couple in the real sense of the word.

You'll be able to say to each other, "Look, we made this happen. We had faith, and because of our faith we've been rewarded with more faith."

As I mentioned in the last chapter, faith is like a muscle. The more you use it, the stronger it gets.

The Stages of Love

Most relationships begin with a burst of inspiration, and then proceed to a second stage marked by frustration and disappointment. The second stage is ordinarily difficult, but you have to get through it to stage three before you really become a couple.

This basic three-step pattern of inspiration, disappointment, and eventual creative mastery seems to be part of the blueprint for human life. Moses famously received two tablets from God on Mount Sinai, but then smashed them after seeing the children of Israel worshipping the golden calf. Tradition teaches that the first tablets were magical, having been carved by God.

The inspiration stage of a romantic relationship is also magical. But it's a gift one hasn't yet earned. One way or another, every relationship ends up breaking its first set of tablets.

Moses ultimately receives a second set of tablets, but they aren't as magical as the first ones. Moses has to cut them with his own hands. But they're good enough for the purpose.

Like Moses, every couple has to cut its second set of tablets by hand. They may not be quite as beautiful as the first set, but they're more authentically yours.

Under One Roof

After months of searching, Emily and Sam find a small one-bedroom apartment on the Upper West Side that they both like, and they nervously both sign their names to the lease.

There are some minor disappointments the first few weeks—such as when they go looking for a couch for their living room and discover they hate each other's taste in furniture. But after a few weeks of serious looking all over town, they find a couch that both of them feel they can live with.

That seems like a good sign. They have sex on the new couch the day it gets delivered. Emily figures that even though neither of them really loves the couch, at least they love each other.

The next Sunday, Emily is reading in the bedroom and Sam comes in to ask her whether she'd mind if he went to the gym before dinner.

It occurs to her that Sam always does this. He always asks like he needs her permission.

For some reason, this gets on her nerves.

That night, Sam seems more hesitant in bed with her. That gets on her nerves too. Sam must notice something is wrong—because midway through intercourse he suddenly loses his erection. Emily tells him it's okay. She's kind of tired anyway.

But inside she starts to feel afraid again, and they start to have sex less and less.

Emily refuses to watch another relationship go down the tubes.

She insists they see a therapist right away—and after a little Google searching they find their way to me.

~~

The first time I see Emily and Sam together, they seem an odd match. An anxious, pale young woman wearing a sweater and thick glasses, and a tanned, athletic-looking young man in a lavender polo shirt. They say they want help with their communication, and with the fact that they've nearly stopped having sex.

It's common for couples to complain about lack of communication. But the reality is usually they've been communicating quite well—just not with words—and that neither of them likes the communications they're getting.

"Do you remember when the trouble started?" I ask.

"I think it was a few weeks after we moved in together," Sam says. "Right after we bought that awful couch. That's when Emily started getting annoyed at me."

"I remember it was when you stopped wanting sex."

Sam looks exasperated. "I never stopped wanting sex. It just started to feel so awkward, and you seemed so annoyed."

Emily is about to argue with him, but she decides not to. She takes a deep breath and lets Sam's words sink in. Maybe she *has* been feeling annoyed with him.

"I remember one time," she says. "You asked me if it was okay if you went to the gym before dinner. For some reason that rubbed me the wrong way."

"I remember that too," says Sam.

"In my family," says Emily, "if a man wants to go somewhere, he doesn't ask anyone's permission."

Sam takes a deep breath. "In my family, you're *supposed* to ask. It's called being polite."

"I *can't imagine* my father or any of my brothers asking permission like that. It's not masculine."

Sam takes another deep breath. "Where I come from, it's considered masculine to treat people with respect."

"Well, it doesn't feel masculine to me," she says. "It turns me off."

Identifications

Harriet Lerner in *The Dance of Anger* makes the point that when a couple argues, they often have no idea what they're actually fighting about. Emily and Sam aren't really fighting about Sam's masculinity. They're really fighting about whether there's any hope for them as a couple.

Emily is scared that maybe they're too different. And for some reason she's doing the same thing she did to her first husband—making him feel unaccepted, which if she keeps it up will probably end up driving him away and confirming her fear that the relationship was never meant to be.

Why in the world would Emily want to do this? It's complicated, and we'll talk about it in Chapter 17.

According to Lerner, sometimes it's not simply that you don't know what you're fighting *about*. Sometimes you have no idea who you're fighting *with*.

In this case, the real battle seems to be inside Emily's head.

We spoke in the last chapter about introjects. Introjects are a common way we remember important people from childhood. Another way is to *identify* with them—to take on their qualities until we actually resemble them in some fashion.

There are positive and negative identifications, just like there are positive and negative introjects. One way the human race survives is because people identify with the good parts of their parents. They pass the good stuff on to the next generation.

But most people also identify with things they *hated* about their parents. The reasons are often obscure, but I think most often it falls under the category of "identifying with the aggressor."

"I don't know if you noticed it," Emily says when I see her alone a week later, "but in your office last week when I was complaining about Sam, I found myself smiling. I couldn't figure out why."

I tell her I hadn't noticed that.

"It was so strange," she says. "Here I was criticizing him, and something inside of me seemed—I don't know—*happy* about it.

"Then I noticed the same thing at home," she says. "Sam was being his usual overconsiderate self. I told him he was irritating me. And there I was—smiling again.

"Then all of a sudden it hit me. It wasn't pleasure. It was *relief*. I thought, 'Thank God it's *him* getting criticized. *Thank God it's not me.*'"

"A lot of people have that experience," I say. "Was there ever someone in your life whose criticism absolutely terrified you?"

"I guess that would be my father," she says. "He could be very harsh. When I was little I'd do anything not to have him criticize me."

"I think when you criticize Sam, you're identifying with your father. We all like to identify with people in power. It's a lot safer."

"My father's a scientist too," she says. "We collaborate sometimes."

"How does your father feel about Sam? Does he like him?"

"Actually, yes. But I'm always expecting he won't. I don't know why."

"Probably because the father in your head is a lot more judgmental than your actual father ever was, even on his worst days."

"Is there anything we can do about the father in my head?"

"That might take a little time. For now, let's just keep a close watch on him. Let me know if he causes any trouble."

Another Turning Point

One day Emily and Sam are at lunch with Emily's parents, and the conversation turns to science. Sam, who admittedly knows very little about science, says something totally ignorant. Emily looks warily over to her father, who raises his eyebrows but says nothing.

After lunch, Emily comes over to where her father is reading the paper. "Dad," she says, "I really appreciated your not correcting Sam at lunch."

Her father is quiet for a moment. "I didn't want to make him feel bad."

"Well, I just wanted to say how much I appreciated it."

It's a tiny exchange of words, but for Emily it's significant. She feels proud that she had the courage to speak to her father in this way.

It's also nice to feel protective of Sam. Somehow Emily feels more kindly toward Sam when she's worried that her father might hurt him.

Emily sits down next to her father, relishing the moment. "Sam is a good man," she says.

"I agree."

"Thanks for being patient with him."

"You didn't think I would be?"

"Sometimes you can be pretty judgmental."

Emily sees her father stiffen a bit—then relax.

"I know," he says, and puts down his paper. "I used to be much worse."

"I remember that," she says. She reaches over on the couch and gives him a hug.

"You're a good man too," she tells him. "I'm lucky to have both of you."

Triangles

Bowen taught that relationships between two people were inherently unstable, and that human society tended to be composed not of pairs but of triangles. Bowen might have pointed to the presence of a triangle involving Sam, Emily, and Emily's father.

Sam provides a safe haven for Emily when she's frustrated with her father, since he's more easygoing and less judgmental. But Emily always feels tempted to run back to the safety of her father introject.

That's not really such a safe spot though, since he's a rather scary introject. Actually neither position in the triangle feels particularly safe, which is one reason Emily feels so anxious most of the time.

That night, Emily tells Sam about her conversation with her father. She's still enjoying that nice protective feeling toward Sam. She climbs on top of him, straddles his waist with her legs, and tells him to lie still while she looks into his eyes. Then Emily asks Sam to look into *her* eyes.

"What do you see?" she asks him.

"Courage," he says. "It looks good on you."

Sam kisses Emily's face, then he lifts her higher and kisses her deeply between her breasts. Soon they are making love and she is crying again.

Sam holds her close and lets her cry. It's been an exhausting few weeks.

Emily is glad she's feeling stronger again. She knows that this good, strong feeling won't always be there. But at least she knows where to find it, and that gives her hope that she'll be able to get it back.

Over time Emily's confidence grows, and she spends more time protecting Sam than attacking him. She discovers that this is not as dangerous a situation as she thought, and the father in her head becomes like one of those monsters under the bed from childhood— not so scary once you're older.

When two people become a couple, there are often many such monsters under the bed. If you face them together, this can be a potent source of faith.

~~~

The first time Emily tells Sam he's not being masculine enough, it confuses him. But after a while he starts to stand his ground. He tells her he won't tolerate being criticized like that anymore.

Emily is relieved. She realizes that all her life she's wanted someone to stand up to her father. When Sam stands up to the *father inside her*, this helps Emily to do so as well.

It feels like a kind of secular exorcism, trying to cast out the father inside her. Emily hates that it's such a slow process. She wishes someone could just come in waving a cross and chanting in Latin and she'd be cured for good.

One day Sam is going out to the gym, and again he asks Emily if she's okay with it. The whole thing still strikes her as very weird.

"You know," she says, "Dad and I still don't like it when you ask permission like that."

"You can both kiss my ass," he answers.

She laughs.

Sons and Lovers

Adam sits in my leather chair, his hands gripping the armrests. Seth sits across from him on the couch. It's the first time I've met Seth.

As you'll recall from Chapter 12, Adam thinks Seth is too feminine. When Adam told me he wanted to come in with Seth today to talk about this, I worried how Seth might react.

Turns out I needn't have worried. Seth isn't having any of it.

"It's all bullshit," says Seth, turning to me. "I think Adam has a problem with his mother."

Adam crosses his arms. "What's wrong with my mother?"

"I watch her sometimes—the way she moves. She has no confidence in herself as a woman. How's she going to help you be confident as a gay man?"

Adam makes a face.

"You're missing one of the great things about being gay," Seth says.

"You don't have that incestuous thing with your mother. You can relax and enjoy each other."

"My mother and I enjoy each other."

"Not the way I'm talking about."

"She accepts me."

"Yeah, but can she just *enjoy* you?"

Seth thinks some more. "When you told her you were gay, she probably went and asked her therapist how to feel about it."

Adam smiles. "Yeah, I bet that's exactly what she did."

Seth thinks for a moment. "I wish you'd just let *me* enjoy you," he says.

Adam looks uncomfortable. "I can't," he says.

"I know," says Seth.

Seth reaches over and roughs up Adam's hair—which Adam doesn't like but under the circumstances deems it wise to tolerate.

Months go by, and I see them together now and then, when they're in New York. Adam says he's starting to see Seth's point of view.

Maybe it would have been different when he was young and just discovering he was different, if his mother *had* just enjoyed him. But Adam finds it hard to imagine that happening back then. The world was such a different place.

Adam finally decides to talk with his mother. He asks her whether she ever noticed that he was different from other boys. She says it crossed her mind, but back then people didn't get into their children's business like they do now.

She says she does wish she'd been able to enjoy him more, just as he was. But that would have taken more confidence in herself than she had back then. She says she thinks *her* mother never had much confidence in herself either. Maybe that got passed down.

Adam's mother tells him she's glad he decided to speak with her about this, and how proud she is of the man he's become. It's an emotional moment for both of them.

Seth and Adam do get married. Adam still feels uneasy sometimes when he thinks Seth isn't acting masculine enough—but he says it doesn't feel like such a big deal now.

Sometimes Adam feels a softness for Seth that he knows is a reaching out to something within himself. Once in a while, he even feels a sense of kindness toward the shy boy he used to be—and in some ways still is.

15

Can Sex Survive Monogamy?

Monogamy can develop your capacity for love, including erotic love. But that doesn't happen automatically. It requires commitment, luck, self-awareness, and the ability not to panic when you don't feel desire.

"My experience indicates that most people become infatuated or fall in love with others an average of six times in the course of a long marriage."
—AVODAH OFFIT, *THE SEXUAL SELF*

It's seven thirty in the morning on a beautiful spring day, and I'm walking crosstown toward Central Park on my way to work. In a few hours the streets will be crowded with tourists. But for now it's mostly just working people like myself, students waiting for a school bus, people walking their dogs.

Arriving at my office just off Central Park, I pause for a moment as the air fills with lilac and honeysuckle. A paved path leads somewhere into shadow beneath the trees. The woods beckon with the promise of spring and the scent of things in bloom. But I have a busy day ahead.

I open the street door to my office. I take one last good look at the brightening sky over my shoulder, and head inside.

The Call of the Wild

Glancing at my inbox, I notice an email from Emily asking if she can see me today.

I haven't seen her in a decade and a half. There's an hour later this afternoon that I was going to use to clear my desk. I offer it to her and she says she'll take it.

I find her in the waiting room doing work on her laptop. She's letting her straight hair go gray, but otherwise she looks much the same.

Emily tells me that she and Sam are still together. They have a son who's now fourteen. She's the head of her department now and runs a big research operation. She says she still loves her job but wishes she didn't have to travel so much.

She looks around my office nostalgically, then gets down to business.

"Here's the problem," she says. "There's someone else—another man—and I need to figure out what to do before it gets out of hand."

"Have you slept with him?"

"No, but I really want to. I'm fifty years old, and I've never met anyone who attracts me so strongly. You're going to think this is crazy, but I don't want to die without having had sex with him at least once."

It turns out he's a fellow scientist in Seattle—about the same age as Emily—an important person in their field, also married with kids. They often share a podium at meetings, and the last few times they've ended up having dinner together afterward. Something is clearly heating up.

I always counsel my married patients to avoid secluding themselves at a restaurant with someone they're attracted to. Sharing food together is part of the primate mating ritual.

"The last time, he and I ended up talking in the hotel restaurant until close to midnight," she says. "I could feel myself lubricating. Thank God it was a big hotel and our floors had separate elevators."

"Have you been emailing each other?"

"I try not to, she says, looking away. It's way too distracting. But sometimes it's hard to resist."

"When are you going to see him next?" I ask.

"There's a meeting in mid-May."

I do a quick calculation of how many weeks that is from now. Not that many.

"How are things with Sam?"

"Okay, I guess. But it's a long time since there's been any real passion between us."

"Why? What's wrong?"

"Nothing really. Sex with Sam just feels like the same thing, over and over again."

Emily blushes, and rebuttons a stray cuff. "Monogamy isn't natural, is it?" she asks.

"No, not really."

"Then why are we supposed to be monogamous, if it's not natural?" She looks away distractedly. I sense she's not really looking for an answer.

"You want advice?" I ask.

"Will it hurt?"

"Probably."

She laughs.

"Don't do it," I tell her. "Don't have dinner with him alone again. Just order room service and take a nice bath. Masturbate, if you want to. But don't do it."

"Why not? A lot of my friends are having affairs. They seem fine."

"This sounds impulsive."

"Maybe I could use a little impulsive right now."

"I think the guilt would drive you crazy. Just enjoy the fact that this other man turns you on. It's just a feeling. Don't let it distract you."

She says she'll think about that.

A Problem as Old as Humankind

Your sexual self doesn't understand the whole monogamy thing at all. Sometimes it just wants what it wants, and there's no reasoning with it.

Strict sexual monogamy is a fairly recent development in human history. We've been a pair-bonded species for millions of years, but sexually exclusive long-term relationships are a relatively new idea.

If you're like most people, your sexual self would love to have it both ways. It likes the security of being exclusive, but once in a while it wouldn't mind some action on the side.

This problem is as old as humankind, and there's no one answer to it.

Not everyone opts for monogamy. It's a choice you make. But if you've decided to be each other's exclusive lovers for life—whether because of your love for each other, your religious beliefs, or other practical considerations—then sooner or later you'll need to know what to do when your sexual self gets restless and wants to try something new.

The first thing is to be firm but gentle and tell yourself "no." In the parenting books this is called "setting limits."

There's nothing bad about wanting what you want. You just can't have it. People who set reasonable limits for themselves tend to be happier than people who don't.

The Bible says, "Thou shalt not covet." But what does that mean?

Not coveting means knowing there are some things you have a right to possess, and other things you don't have a right to possess. Not coveting is like not stealing. They're both about setting good limits.

Again, though, this is assuming you're serious about monogamy. These days there are lots of other options (see Notes). But most people I see in my office still want to be monogamous.

Even more important, they want their *partners* to be monoga-

mous. So it seems only fair to hold themselves to the same standard.

Love and Loss

Several weeks later Emily emails me asking for another appointment, and I arrange to see her later that week.

"I took your advice," she says. "I just ordered room service and
took a bath. I masturbated like crazy that night, but when I got on
the plane to go home I knew I'd done the right thing. The peace of
mind was worth it."

A thought occurs to me.

"Have you ever found yourself this turned on by a man before?"
I ask.

"No, I don't think so."

"That must mean something. What else is going on in your life
these days?"

"Nothing out of the ordinary. We both work too hard, but we're
okay with that. Sam and my son are doing all right." She thinks
for a moment. "The only bad thing is my father's been sick."

"I'm sorry to hear that."

"He has heart problems, and he's been in the hospital a lot." She
buttons the cuff of her sleeve. "Do you think that might be relevant?"

"It *does* sound like a serious loss."

She grimaces. "Hey, he's not dead yet."

"It's still a loss. The erotic mind doesn't handle loss very well. I
wonder if some of this longing you've been feeling might be your
sexual self trying to cheer you up."

"Why couldn't I just cheer myself up with Sam?"

"You mentioned sex with him hasn't been very satisfying."

She thinks for a moment.

"That happens with all couples, right?"

"I think this is something more specific. There's always been some kind of emotional triangle between you and Sam and your father. After your father got sick, I wonder if you unconsciously looked for someone to replace him in that triangle. I don't think it's an accident that you got horny for another scientist."

"That's deep," she says. "But it makes sense."

"You want advice?"

She gives me a look and a smile. "Take another bath and masturbate?"

"No, silly. Let's get you and Sam back together."

She presses her lips together and looks grim. "We've tried everything," she says. "Toys, porn, sex dates. Nothing seems to work."

"Those things are mostly useless," I tell her. "Let's have you try something different."

What Not to Do When You Lose Desire

If you look on the web for advice on how to bring back desire, the first suggestion you'll usually get is to put more novelty and adventure back into your sex life. Novelty and adventure—whether in the form of sex toys, fetish props, sexy videos, or sexy dates and destinations—are consumer society's answer to sexual boredom.

But these things seldom do the trick. Working hard to keep your sexual self happy can be like trying to keep a child entertained. Long term, you're not likely to make the child any happier. Usually you'll just end up exhausting yourself.

Worse still, if your drawer is full of sex toys but you're still feeling unsatisfied in bed, this can leave you feeling even more discouraged than when you started out.

If you have a reasonably good erotic connection together, erotic novelty can sometimes be fun. But if you're looking for something to *restore* your desire for each other, then I wouldn't jump to novelty as the answer.

Sure, go ahead and try those handcuffs if you like. But unless you're fundamentally kinky, don't bet on novelty and adventure to keep desire alive.

So . . . What's the Alternative?

All right, you say. So how *can* you keep desire alive?

Here's the secret: *You can't.*

This is important.

Desire comes and goes many times over the course of a long-term erotic relationship. You can't control desire, any more than you can control the whims of a child.

Desire is nice, but you don't *need* desire to have good sex. One reason so many people end up having bad sex is because they try to force desire.

If you need to cultivate a sense of adventure in order to keep yourself interested in your partner, that's forcing desire.

If you need to watch porn to feel like getting it on, that's forcing desire.

If you're making "sex dates" just to have sex, without feeling anything, that's forcing desire.

Try to force desire, and sooner or later you'll have a rebellion on your hands.

~~

If you're like most people, you don't just want sex to satisfy you. You want sex to *inspire* you. But it's crucial when you go looking for erotic inspiration that you first look within yourself.

If you're not feeling desire, you can't just make a date to have sex and expect it to help. But you *can* make a date to just lie naked in bed together, with each of you having no agenda other than to pay close attention, without judgment, to what you're actually feeling.

Carmen from Chapter 6 did this when she lay in bed with Scott and just listened to the silence. Marnie from Chapter 10 did this when she spent time in bed with Tom and told him all about her sadness and frustration. These experiences weren't in themselves erotic, but they gave Carmen and Marnie's sexual selves a clear message of acceptance and understanding.

Once your sexual self feels accepted and understood, then it can calm down. Once it no longer feels forced or manipulated, then it can act on its own free will.

When you first become a couple, you spend lots of time lost in the moment. That's what arousal does to you. It puts you in the moment.

When you've been together a while, that kind of moment is something you have to cultivate. It doesn't usually happen on its own.

But that moment of connection can be more important than whether or not you end up having sex. In that moment there is a stillness that once you make contact with it can nourish your erotic life together for a long while.

Sex in Midlife

Many couple's capacity for channeling erotic energy tends to diminish a bit in midlife. As a result, being sexual together can start to feel awkward.

When this happens, the most important thing is not to panic. Your erotic mind is not a servant that just shows up to work every day. Its nature is freer and more creative.

By midlife, most couples should spend some time opening up together before engaging in any serious lovemaking. One of the biggest mistakes I see midlife couples make is to go to bed and try to have sex immediately, without first taking the time to open up. That can be a surefire recipe for bad sex.

Here's the basic Two-Step recipe I recommend for most couples. Feel free to modify it to suit your needs:

Step One

Spend some time in bed doing nothing together. Most couples prefer to be naked, but do whatever makes you feel most comfortable.

If you like, you can talk about whatever is on your mind—good, bad, or indifferent. Anything at all. It doesn't have to be erotic. But keep it simple. No big discussions.

When you feel you've talked as much as you need or want to, see if you can give yourselves permission to just be together quietly, doing nothing.

With eyes open or closed, see where your awareness and your senses take you. You may want to notice your breathing, the temperature of your skin, the way your body presses against the mattress.

This might not feel erotic at all at first. That's fine. Sometimes you might just feel a little quieter. But in time that quiet can be the soil from which arousal grows.

Feel free to get creative with Step One. I've known several couples where one partner's best Step One was just to complain for five minutes while the other partner gave them their full attention.

Step Two

At some point during Step One you may notice feeling aroused. If arousal happens, just enjoy it for its own sake. Don't worry about your partner. They can take care of themselves.

Arousal isn't all-or-none. Sometimes it can be rather subtle—a private, inward thing. Take your time.

Eventually you may want to communicate to your partner about your arousal, in whatever way you like. A little talking can be quite helpful at this point. Most couples don't talk enough during sex.

Don't worry about arousal. Let your arousal take care of *you*. If you can, just be a passenger and let it take you wherever it wants.

Cat, Cow, Cobra, Child

The next weekend morning, by mutual agreement, Emily and Sam go back to bed after brushing their teeth. They lie quietly next to each other naked under the covers—each paying attention to their breathing, the temperature, the way their bodies press against the mattress. There are a few giggles at first, but then a stillness settles over the bedroom.

"I miss the old days," says Sam, "when you used to tell me things that scared you."

"Me too," says Emily. "I guess I ran out of things that scared me."

"Is anything scaring you now?"

"I'm scared this isn't going to work," says Emily.

"Me too," says Sam.

"I want to feel you again," Emily says.

Emily tells Sam to lie on his stomach. She takes one of his hands and explores it with her fingers. It's strange just to lie here with nothing to do but experience her own body, and his. She strokes his arm, then his shoulder, then runs the backs of her fingernails across his back and down his other arm. She feels the tiniest bit aroused. Then it passes.

"I like this," she says.

"Can I turn over?" he asks.

"No, not yet. I want to take my time."

It's nice to be in charge, she thinks. Not to have to worry whether she's getting turned on or not. Or whether she's wet enough, or whether to go get lubricant. Just to be in the moment. Emily realizes she hasn't been in the moment for a long time.

Emily wonders whether it might help to get her body moving. She gets up and straddles Sam's waist, raises herself up on her knees, stretches her arms high in the air for a bit, then puts her palms down on either side of Sam's head.

Planted there on her knees and palms, she rounds her back and lets her head hang. What do they call this in yoga? Oh, yeah—"the cat pose." Then she lifts her head as high as it will go, letting her back slouch down—"the cow."

Cat. Cow. She alternates them a few more times. Her body feels more alive now.

Emily wonders whether she's aroused or just happy to be moving her body. She raises her chest and tilts her head back—"the cobra"— or about as close to a cobra as you can do on a grown man's back.

She lowers herself down again and lets her breasts graze his back. Mmm, definitely a little aroused. She sits back on Sam's tailbone and lets it support her weight. She leans forward and drapes herself on his back. She's sweating a little but it feels good.

Breathing deeply, Emily rests her head to one side on his shoulder and inhales the scent of his hair—"the child."

Sam keeps very still. "Are you doing yoga on my back?" he asks.

"Uh-huh."

"You're blowing my mind. Tell me when I can turn over, okay?"

Emily continues in the child pose, letting her muscles go all loose on Sam's back.

"You may turn over now, my man," she says.

Sam takes her face in his hands, just like he used to do when they first met.

"Ready for more Step Two?" she asks.

"I thought you'd never ask."

Mindfulness, Heartfulness, and Prayer

Most couples crave erotic inspiration. Happily, that's something most couples can achieve. Not by becoming more masterful lovers, but by making eros an instrument of sanctification and peace.

"In my opinion, there are two things that can absolutely not be carried to the screen: the realistic presentation of the sexual act and praying to God."
—ORSON WELLES

Emily and Sam lie together afterward.

"What'd you think?"

"I loved it. I didn't have to think about getting turned on. I just let it happen."

"That was a nice touch there—with the yoga," he says.

Emily knows it probably would never have occurred to her to try doing yoga on Sam's back if she hadn't just done the mindfulness practice with him. But once she'd been in the moment, it seemed so obvious that her body needed to move and stretch. She hasn't really lived in her body for a long time.

"I wish we'd got that on video," he says, laughing.

She punches his shoulder. He laughs harder.

Then something occurs to Emily. She thinks for a minute.

"You know, you always do that. You always make some playful comment."

"Is that bad?"

"It throws me off balance sometimes. I used to like it, because it kept things light. But right now I just want to be serious with you."

Sam thinks for a minute. "I like that you're telling me that," he says.

"You sure?"

"Yeah. It reminds me of our first year together. Do you remember, you used to be so anxious and overwhelmed and the only thing that seemed to help was to tell me things you didn't want to tell me?"

"I'd forgotten all about that."

There's something else Sam wants to talk about—especially now that they've just had reasonably good sex and Emily seems to want to relate on a more serious level.

Ever since the summer, Emily has had a faraway look, and Sam has wondered if she's really there. He takes a deep breath. Here it comes.

"For a while recently, I've thought you might be cheating on me."

Now it's Emily's turn to take a deep breath.

"For a while, I wanted to."

"Did you?"

Emily shakes her head.

"What stopped you?"

"Dr. Snyder told me not to. It was worse than you knew. I had no inspiration for us anymore. Everything we tried just seemed to backfire."

Sam is quiet, taking this all in.

"He told me the trouble was we were trying to force desire—you know, with porn and everything. He said if you try to force desire, you can easily end up with a rebellion on your hands. I'm pretty sure that's what happened to me."

Emily thinks some more. "The first year we were together, it felt so natural to get excited. I don't mean just wet. I mean silly and happy and really wanting it.

"Then all of a sudden it just didn't happen like that anymore. Dr. Snyder says that happens to a lot of couples. It's a sign that they need to spend more time together in bed doing nothing at all—like we did this morning. But instead, most couples start trying to force things.

"It's like a fantasy, or a vibrator. It's fine if you're already excited, and that gets you higher or takes you over the top. But it shouldn't be your foundation together."

Emily thinks some more. "Do you think you can forgive me?" she says.

"For what?" says Sam. "You didn't do anything."

"For wanting to."

"I'll think about it," he says, smiling, and pulls her close.

Emily peels his hand away from her body. "No. Serious, remember?"

"Okay," he says. "I can do serious."

"Now, can you forgive me?"

Sam thinks about it. "I still don't think it's necessary," he says. "But if you need me to, then sure—I forgive you."

Sam is quiet again for a moment. Emily watches his face.

"It's good to have you back," he says.

More Than Two

I see Emily and Sam a few times after that. Then they go away on vacation, and I don't hear from Emily again until mid-September when she emails me asking for an appointment alone.

"I have a special favor to ask," she says when I come to get her in the waiting room. "Can we go to the park instead? I don't want to waste this day sitting inside."

Ordinarily I'd say no. As a therapist, it's part of your job to maintain the boundaries of the treatment. But something in her expression tells me this is important. I look on my schedule to make sure I don't have anyone scheduled after her.

Even though the summer is winding down, there are still tourist buses lined up on Seventy-Second Street and crowds of people moving back and forth near the park. We make our way past the souvenir stands, take a left at Strawberry Fields, and walk down the steep road to the lake.

"Sam took me out in one of those little boats on our first date," she says as we look for a clean bench.

"How was it?"

"Oh, you know. It was how it always is when you've just gotten three years of federal research funding and this really handsome guy seems interested in you. It was good."

"Are things still all right with the two of you?"

"More than all right," she says.

Emily looks out at the water. "Look, I need to ask you something. I'm still in touch with my man from Seattle. Turns out he's a lot like me. Reasonably happy marriage, nice kids. Here's the thing: I still desire him fiercely. Do you think there could ever be a way for that to work out?"

"You mean leaving Sam?"

"No. I mean having them both."

Emily brushes back her hair. "Look, we're all in our fifties. Why can't we just share?"

It feels weird being out in the park like this talking about wife-swapping. I half expect the state medical board to come arrest me.

"What if Sam asked you to share him with another woman?"

"That would be hard. But lots of things are hard. Like leaving home. It's hard, but you do it because it's necessary. You might be homesick at first, but eventually you're glad you took the leap."

"So sharing partners is the next leap?"

"Why not? I think the only thing that keeps us all monogamous is because we think that's what our neighbors are doing. Are you and your wife monogamous?"

"We're religious. It's a commandment."

"Do you really think God wants us to be monogamous?"

"I think He wants us not to covet what doesn't belong to us."

"If my neighbor lets me drive his Ferrari and I take it out for a bit and then give it back to him, is that coveting?"

"People aren't cars. They don't exist to satisfy us."

"Hopefully he'd get something out of it too."

"Do you really think you'd do this?"

Emily smooths out her dress.

"I guess not," she says. "Not unless I sat down with Sam and he agreed to it—because who wants to go sneaking around? And I'd probably want to wait until our son was married—because who wants pervy in-laws? And by then, we'll probably all be so old that it won't be worth the trouble."

We both laugh.

"Are you really religious?" she asks.

"I do my best to be."

"Why?"

"Lots of reasons. Mostly because at a certain point in my life I needed a relationship with God."

"Is it weird, being religious and a sex therapist?"

"No, it's nice. They're both about relationships."

Sex and Religion

When my beloved first stands before me naked, all open to my sight, there is a feeling throughout the whole of me; awe. Why?

If sex is no more than an instinct, why don't I simply feel horny or hungry? Such simple hunger would be quite sufficient to insure the propagation of the species.

Why awe? Why should sex be complicated by reverence?

—M. SCOTT PECK, *THE ROAD LESS TRAVELED*

Why should sex be complicated by reverence? Good question. Many years ago, M. Scott Peck described his encounter with religious awe in the form of a woman's naked body. Peck's sense of wonder at the miracle of sexuality resonated with many people's intuition that sex had a religious dimension.

Not many sex writers have dealt with religion, and fewer still have described it in a positive way. That's understandable, considering all the horrible crimes against sexuality that have been committed in the name of religion. But I know I'm not alone in thinking sex and religion must have something important to say to each other.

Today religion is a more forbidden subject than sex. Many years ago, when I was just starting to think about these issues, I had a patient whom I'd gotten to know very well. I knew what sex positions she preferred, how long it took her to reach orgasm, how often she masturbated, and the content of her sexual fantasies.

At one point—I forget why—I asked her if she ever prayed. She was shocked at the question, and said it was way too personal. I quickly learned that religious questions are very likely to rub patients the wrong way.

That's a shame. Sex and religion are both ultimately about connection, and most truly religious people have a lot of experience with losing their faith and needing to find it again—or at least replenish it.

I think every erotic couple eventually develops a private religion of their own—and every time you make love together you're performing a sacrament within this private religion.

People are diverse in their spiritual inclinations. But I believe most people hunger for sanctity in their lives, and that good lovemaking can help satisfy that hunger.

Mindfulness, Heartfulness, and Prayer

In his book *Mindfulness for Beginners*, Jon Kabat-Zinn notes that the word for "mind" and the word for "heart" are the same in many Asian languages. So "heartfulness" is automatically implied in "mindfulness."

Mindfulness practice is of Indian and East Asian origin. It has no precise Western equivalent.

But I think the Western concept of *prayer* might have some untapped possibilities here.

People tend to associate prayer with asking for things. But theologically speaking, that's silly. If there is a God, He surely doesn't need you to ask Him for what you need. He already knows.

A more sensible definition of prayer would involve purposefully clearing away all your other concerns, so you can open yourself up to inspiration.

One mystical notion holds that the blessings for which you pray are already all around you. Prayer is simply creating a proper vessel to receive them.

Lovemaking itself can be a form of prayer. Great sex, like deep prayer, can be an act of surrender—where the erotic energy of the universe fills you up and passes through you, leaving you grateful and fulfilled. But even simple, ordinary good sex can be a sacred act, if done with the right intention.

The Sanctification of the Ordinary

Many sex writers start with an image—an ideal—of human erotic potential. The point of reference is usually sex that is transcendent or extraordinary—what one writer called "peak erotic experiences."

Me, I'm not that interested in my patients' peak experiences. They're nice when they happen, but I don't think they do much to increase your faith.

I believe real faith grows from the sanctification of the ordinary. When as a couple you commit on a regular basis to going to bed early to talk, and perhaps to making love afterward, that's a sanctification of the ordinary.

Back when you started out together, sex was one of the only ways you had of reassuring each other that everything was going to be okay. Holding each other, and being held, helped give you faith.

Now maybe you have other sources of reassurance. Accomplishments, children, or a nice home in a good community. But you keep having sex anyway because it keeps your faith channel open.

The main thing is to start where you are. It has to be honest, or it won't work. Inspiration may come in time. You can't force it. It has its own rhythms, and you have to respect them. "Inspiration exists," said Picasso. "But it has to find you working."

Inspiration exists in sex too—but you have to open yourself up to it.

Getting Practical:
Sex Tune-Ups for Couples

Many years ago, treatment at the Masters and Johnson clinic often started with something called "sensate focus." This involved getting naked and taking turns caressing each other, just for its own sake, without any expectation of turning the other person on—or getting them off.

Couples seemed to like it a lot. It often provided a welcome relief from all the bad sex they'd been having.

During your first few sensate focus sessions, you'd take care to avoid any explicitly erotic places on your partner's body. Then you'd move on to include these sexier parts—but not in the usual goal-oriented way.

Instead, the person doing the touching would simply focus on the experience of touching their partner's body, and the person being touched would just allow them to (unless it became uncomfortable, of course). Nobody had to worry about or take care of anybody else. Which if you've never tried it can be a wonderful kind of freedom.

Sensate focus was extremely popular in its day, and most sex therapists still recommend it. But for some reason most couples these days don't find it so interesting. Maybe it's because our attention spans are shorter. I don't know.

Most people got sensate focus wrong anyway. They'd work hard to give their partner the best touch experience possible. As you know, that kind of generosity is not so erotic. What's worse, it created a demand on the receiver to appreciate the gesture—which of course isn't so erotic either.

The original idea, now generally forgotten, was that both touching and being touched were supposed to be strictly selfish activities. It wasn't so much "giving touch" as "taking touch." As the receiver, you'd know that your partner was enjoying your body selfishly—for their own pleasure. You were free to experience the process in whatever way you liked, without having to worry about them.

As Masters and Johnson continued to prescribe sensate focus to their clients, it gradually became clear to them that the idea of prescribing pleasure at all made no sense, and was all wrong. Pleasure is an emotion, and you can't control emotions.

So in later years the pleasure prescription was withdrawn. Patients would be told to just have the experience, with no expectation at all of whether it would be pleasurable or not.

Unfortunately not much of this was ever written down, and for decades sex therapists have been instructing their patients to "take pleasure" during sensate focus—or even worse, to "pleasure their partners."

A lot of people still benefited from even these misguided attempts at sensate focus. There's nothing wrong with simply giving pleasure or taking pleasure, especially if the alternative is some kind of bad sex. But the technique can do so much more in the right hands.

Recently two former Masters and Johnson staff therapists, Linda Weiner and Constance Avery-Clark, have been leading a movement to educate sex therapists about this more rigorous way to do sensate focus. And as a result, sensate focus seems to be making a comeback.

Part of the field's renewed interest in sensate focus may have to do with the fact that it's essentially a mindfulness practice. If you do it right, sensate focus can be an effective tool for getting into the present moment and getting out of your own way.

As a matter of fact, all of the practical techniques we've discussed along the way—simmering, outercourse, lazy sex, Two-Stepping, sensate focus—can all be mindfulness practices.

Almost anything at all can be a mindfulness practice, if you keep that intention in mind.

Care of the Sexual Soul

One of the great achievements of faith is to enable people who have been starved for love to experience the ordinary erotic pleasure that most people take for granted. And to feel they deserve it.

"If love is a place, even if it's a scary place, I want to live there."

—GLENNON DOYLE, *LOVE WARRIOR*

Sarina and Jo have been together now for many years. As you'll remember, I helped them over a rough patch in their lovemaking in Chapter 12 when they first became a couple.

Sometimes a rough patch like that just needs a little mending and then everything is fine. But often it's a sign of something deeper that will continue to cause trouble until it's finally healed. With Sarina and Jo, it turns out to be the latter.

Sarina and Jo stay together, raise two children, and finally marry once the law permits it. Now they're here to see me again, two attractive professional women in their early fifties, sitting side by side again on my couch and telling me about how Sarina seems to have lost all interest in sex.

The problem isn't really a new one. It's been brewing for years.

We spend some time catching up, and I get to see pictures of their children on Sarina's iPhone. Then Jo turns to Sarina and asks if she can tell me the whole story.

"Do I have a choice?" says Sarina, looking grim. "Sure."

"To tell you the truth," says Jo, "Sarina's sex drive has always been weirdly passive-aggressive. We'll plan a weekend away, just the two of us—and then the day we're supposed to leave Sarina picks a fight with me and says she has no interest in sex the whole time we're away."

"Is that accurate?" I ask Sarina.

"Pretty much," she says.

"It's like when we were first dating," says Jo, "and you ditched me at that party—"

"Do we have to talk about that?"

"I think it's relevant."

Jo turns to me. "We spend all day together, then a couple of drinks later she's making out with my ex."

"I had no idea she was your ex."

"Irrelevant." Jo thinks a moment. "Then miraculously we survive as a couple, and a few months later you bring me into Dr. Snyder's office complaining that I'm not aggressive enough in bed? I mean, get real!"

"And how is *that* relevant? I thought we were going to talk about the here and now."

"It's all the same. You're always trying to throw me off balance. This not being in the mood for sex now that we're finally empty-nesters is just the latest version."

Enactments

When Sarina and Jo first saw me twenty years ago in Chapter 12, we focused on what Helen Kaplan would have called *immediate causes*. Things that make rational sense, like wanting more passion or more acceptance.

But losing desire just before you're going to leave for a romantic weekend doesn't make any rational sense. Neither does losing desire when your children go off to college—though you could probably invent rationalizations for either one.

When something doesn't make any rational sense, that can be a valuable clue that you're dealing with *remote* causes. Things that, to really understand them, you'd have to go back to your childhood, because they make no sense in the here and now.

I've already told you about introjects and identifications, which in a way are both forms of memory. But there's a third form of memory that I haven't told you about yet that's often a factor in this kind of situation.

This third form of memory is called "enactment." Enactment is when you unconsciously get another person to play a part in a drama that neither you nor they fully understand. (If you understood it, you probably wouldn't need to enact it.)

Enactments are an everyday form of magic. People enact their unconscious fantasies and expectations with the world around them all the time. And the magic is that very often the world plays along.

Someone who was genuinely adored as a child will usually grow up expecting people to adore them. And as if by magic, adoring partners will reliably show up.

Someone who felt unloved, on the other hand, will often be attracted to partners who don't love them. And if by good fortune they meet one who does, they may try very hard to convince them that they shouldn't.

I wouldn't be surprised if Sarina and Jo have been trapped in some kind of enactment since the beginning of their relationship. When you spend the whole day with a new partner and then hook up with someone else that night in full view of your new partner (even if you *don't* know it's her ex), it's a good bet you're enacting something—most often some childhood memory of having been abused, confused, neglected, or otherwise made to feel rejected.

Abuse—whether physical, sexual, or emotional—is usually

something you remember. Neglect tends to be harder to nail down. After all, how can you notice something that never happened?

As my colleague Ruth Cohn points out, when someone who didn't get enough attention, respect, or love growing up is asked about what might have happened in their childhood, often the answer is "nothing." That answer is sometimes unwittingly accurate.

To heal from trauma, you have to find a way to grieve. But how can you properly grieve what you never knew? People who've been neglected often enact it—by neglecting their partners, or by managing to get themselves neglected. Most often both.

There's the so-called Golden Rule that everybody knows: "Do unto others as you would have them do unto you." Then there's the *real* Golden Rule: "Do unto others what *was* done to you."

That *real* Golden Rule is an important one to remember.

From Nothing to Something

"I always figured it's because Sarina never had a real bedroom growing up," says Jo.

"Where did you sleep?" I ask Sarina.

"It was part of the den. They fixed it up for me because there weren't enough bedrooms."

"There weren't enough bedrooms because after your parents' divorce your mother remarried right away, and your stepfather had lots of young kids," says Jo.

"You didn't rate getting a bedroom?" I ask.

"My mother was mainly focused on making my stepfather happy. His kids came first."

"Ouch. How about your father?"

"He remarried quickly too, and they started a new family right away. I never really felt welcome there. After a while I just stopped going."

"Sarina," I say, "when you withdraw from Jo, I wonder if you might be trying to let her know how unloved you felt as a child."

"I'm not sure I *felt* unloved as a child."

"What *do* you remember feeling?"

"Not much of anything, really. I thought that was just the way it was."

Jo is listening intently. "Sarina, I just realized something. You weren't just unloved. You never even knew you *deserved* to be loved."

Sarina looks at her. "I'm not sure I *do* know that."

Jo takes Sarina's hand, and strokes it gently. "You poor child."

Sarina starts to cry. "I'm angry that you don't think I know what I'm feeling."

Jo holds her and strokes her hair. "No, babe," she says. "That's not what I meant."

Then Jo thinks again, and pulls back to where she can see Sarina's face.

"Actually," she says, "that's *exactly* what I meant. Sometimes I think you don't have the *foggiest idea* what you're feeling. Every time I try to express love for you, you do something that says, '*Hah!* Do you love *this?*' Our entire relationship you've been trying to convince me that loving you is a bad idea. And you don't even know that's what you're doing."

They sit quietly holding hands on the couch, both crying softly.

I really don't want this just to be about Sarina. There's always another side to these things.

"Jo," I ask, "when Sarina is cold to you, how do you usually react?"

"I just wait for it to pass. It always does, sooner or later. Why?"

"Where'd you get all that patience?"

Sarina joins in. "Probably from having to deal with her mother," she says.

Jo turns to me. "My mother used to be very cold sometimes."

"Like Sarina?"

"Worse. It used to last much longer."

"Was that scary?"

"I think it must have been. I always figured that was just the way it had to be."

Sarina looks up, smiling through her tears. "I guess I'm not the only one who didn't know she deserved better."

The Blank Page

"So what can we do about sex?" Jo asks when all the crying stops.

I ask Sarina if she still has enough energy to talk about this today. She nods, and grabs a few more tissues.

"I think you might have a real opportunity here," I tell them. "I don't think either of you has ever really felt you deserved to feel wanted."

"How do you mean?" asks Jo.

"Sarina, every time Jo wants you, you go cold. Jo, you've just accepted that. I think if either of you really felt you deserved to feel wanted, none of this would have happened."

"So what do we do?" asks Jo.

I explain to them about sensate focus. I tell them I think they'd probably do best with the most rigorous form of it, where each person has an opportunity to "take touch" from the other, selfishly, without the other having to do anything at all except push them away if something really doesn't feel good.

"That sounds kind of artificial," says Sarina.

"It *is* artificial. It's a blank page. You get to write whatever's inside you. The artificiality makes sure nothing gets in your way."

"If our problem is that neither of us feel we deserve to be wanted, wouldn't it just be better to do affirmations or something?" says Jo.

"You could do that, I guess. I don't love affirmations, because half the time you're going to be saying something you don't really feel. Your sexual self is very sensitive to bullshit. It knows when you're feeling it, and when you're not. I like sensate focus better, because you're not *required* to feel anything that you don't really feel."

"I say we give his method a try," says Sarina. "I want to feel what I really feel."

Into the River

Sarina, having lost the coin toss, lies naked in bed on her stomach—head to one side. Jo, having won the coin toss, sits on a chair beside the bed, wondering where to start.

Don't think so much, Jo says to herself. *Just start wherever.*

Jo moves her chair to the foot of the bed, covers Sarina with a blanket, and begins to touch Sarina's feet. She wants to ask Sarina if that feels good, but then she remembers that's not her job now.

Darn, what *is* her job? Oh, yes—now she remembers: to touch, to notice, to feel whatever she feels—without judgment. That sounded easy, but all of a sudden Jo's mind is a jumble of thoughts. *What day is it? Sunday. Busy day at work tomorrow. Am I doing this right? Will this help? Or will we fail at it, and be no better off than before—just more discouraged?*

Jo's back hurts a little. Maybe sit a little straighter. Mmm, that's better. Jo decides to pay attention to her own breathing before going any further. First one breath, then another.

Jo gives Sarina's right foot her full attention. Then each toe, one by one, noting its shape, temperature, how it connects to the foot.

Jo suddenly feels an urge to kiss Sarina's toes. Is that allowed? She plants a small kiss on each one. *That felt good.*

Jo kisses Sarina's toes again, exactly the same way, one after the other.

What am I feeling now? Jo asks herself.

She takes another breath.

Quiet. I feel quiet now.

Is quiet a feeling? she wonders.

At first, Sarina too has trouble with the sheer number of thoughts that crowd her mind.

What am I feeling now? she asks herself. *Self-conscious, mostly. I'm glad I'm on my belly, where it's more protected. But I still feel self-conscious.*

How about now? She thinks. *What am I feeling now?*

The answer surprises her, and makes her unhappy:

Right now, for some reason I'm mostly just feeling terribly sad. It's like Jo is knocking at my feet but there's nobody home. What does she want?

Then she remembers—*it doesn't matter what Jo wants. Jo is responsible for Jo. You just be responsible for you. Why is that so hard to remember? And what is this terrible sadness?*

Wait, she thinks. *Dr. Snyder talked to us about this. What did he say? Something about how it's not the feeling, it's all the panic attached to it. Why am I so afraid of this sadness?*

Sarina decides to be brave and let the feeling of sadness rise up inside her. Soon it's all the way up to her chest, a strong current of sadness.

What if it reaches my mouth? she thinks. *Will I float? Or will I drown?* Sarina feels Jo kissing her toes, and it's as if Jo is urging Sarina to lift her feet off the bottom and find out. When she does, she feels herself lifted up, carried along in the great current of sadness with no idea where it's taking her.

～

Jo kisses Sarina's toes one more time. Her hands move up to the arch and heel of Sarina's foot—then to her ankle, her leg, her knee. Sarina's foot makes contact with Jo's chest.

Mmm, Jo thinks to herself. *That feels good.* She leaves Sarina's foot where it is, and leans into it with her chest—then bends down and plants a soft kiss on Sarina's heel.

Jo feels something familiar rising inside her—something predatory, drunken. Is *this* allowed? She can't remember. *What did*

Dr. Snyder say? Oh, yes. He said if you happen to feel aroused, just let it happen. Just allow it.

How do you just let arousal happen, she wonders, *without* doing anything about it?

Guess I'm about to find out.

Jo lets herself savor the predatory, drunken feeling in silence. Then it passes, leaving Jo feeling happy and relaxed—and strangely satisfied.

Well, that *was interesting. I didn't know arousal could come and go like that.*

Jo drops Sarina's right foot and picks up Sarina's other foot from where it's been lying patiently, waiting its turn.

~~

Sarina drifts along in her river of sadness. The current is warm, and shows no sign of stopping. Sarina feels Jo's chest pressing against her foot—as if Jo is pushing her farther into the current, all the while keeping her steady in the middle of the river.

Sarina suddenly feels shy about all the attention she's getting.

"I'm worried you're getting tired," she says, aloud.

"Just stay with what you're doing," says Jo in a whisper. "I'm taking care of me. You just take care of you. I'll be fine."

Jo's voice sounds calm, assured. The river doesn't seem quite so sad now.

Jo is beside her now on the bed, stroking the small of Sarina's back.

I'd like this to go on for a long time, Sarina thinks.

"Are you sure you're not getting tired?" she says aloud to Jo.

"Very sure. Just stay with it, Sarina."

My name, thinks Sarina. *She said my name. Why does that make me feel so emotional?*

Yes, Yes, a Thousand Times Yes

Sarina never figures out exactly why it feels so emotional during sensate focus when Jo says her name. But for a while she's desperate to hear it. It's like needing to be kissed, held, loved, noticed, paid attention to. A thousand times a day still wouldn't be enough.

For a while Sarina wants to do sensate focus every day—as if her life depends on it. Sometimes she floats in the river. Sometimes she sits on the shore, just watching it go by.

Many times it's terribly lonely and sad. Memories come to the surface, scary memories. Her parents' divorce, her mother's remarriage, and Sarina as a child, lost in the shuffle. No one ever taught her it was okay to be sad or scared. A lifetime of sadness and grief flows into the river.

Then day by day the grass on the banks turns greener and more lush, and eventually the river empties into a bright lake. Sarina imagines she and Jo are rolling on a blanket by the lake. Sarina feels Jo getting aroused, and she thinks, "Yes, take me. Take all you want. There's enough in me for everyone, and it's all good."

Not many people have as powerful an experience with sensate focus as Sarina does. But every once in a while you meet someone like Sarina who says, "Yes, that's what I need—for a long, long time, until I'm all filled up."

18

Childhood's End

What's the purpose of erotic love in a lasting relationship?
To fill you up, to inspire you, and to nourish your faith.
Everything else is secondary.

"All the rivers run into the sea; yet the sea is not full; unto
the place from whence the rivers come, thither they return
again. . . . The thing that hath been, it is that which shall be;
and that which is done is that which shall be done: and there is
nothing new under the sun."
—ECCLESIASTES 1:7–9

On the internet, for a while, there's a video of a young couple making love. It's not a pornographic video, but I think most people
would find it arousing.

The video is for a brief time part of an advertisement for a piece
of furniture—a narrow, leather chaise longue intended for Tantra
practice.

Tantra is an Indian tradition that's at least a thousand years old,
and in some respects much older. As you may know, part of this
tradition involves sex.

~

The couple in the video are both young and quite beautiful.
They could easily be a couple of college students who just came in

from playing tennis and suddenly decided to take off their clothes in the middle of the living room. He's lying back on the leather chair, his feet flat on the floor. She's astride him, facing away.

The chair is low enough that her feet touch the floor easily, and she keeps rising from the balls of her feet—rocking intently—her eyes half closed. Unlike in conventional pornography, she is wearing no makeup. Her hair needs combing, and her face is quite flushed. Her attention is turned inward—her expression taut, ecstatic, saintly.

But her body's exuberant energy is like that of any child on a playground. Her breasts are in constant motion. For the first time, you understand why Solomon in Song of Songs compares his beloved's breasts to "twin fawns of a gazelle, grazing among the lilies." They are that alive.

She is a magnificent sight—an erotic stone sculpture from an Indian temple, come to life.

But what's most striking is the Indian music in the background. It's slow, sad, and out of pace with the frenzied action on the screen. An older woman's voice chanting in a foreign tongue. Her voice is plaintive, full of longing or grief.

How strange, you think. Such slow, sad music. Why such sadness?

～

You look again a few months later, and the video is gone. Now there are other videos of the same couple, but they're not the same.

The young woman's hair is more carefully done now, and the flush is gone from her face. Makeup, no doubt. The old, keening music has been replaced by something more upbeat.

But the old music still haunts you. The song seemed ancient. It seemed to span years, centuries, millennia. You couldn't understand the words, but they seemed to speak of transience and loss—about things that bloom brightly for a day and then are gone.

"Enjoy this now," the ancient music seemed to say to the young couple. "But know that you are only this year's flowers. Soon the cycle will repeat again, exactly the same—but without you."

You imagine an endless procession of such couples going down through the centuries—the same scene, over and over again.

It's a vision we Westerners aren't accustomed to. We're used to thinking that the world has a direction—that it's steadily moving toward something better. The more ancient idea that "there is nothing new under the sun" doesn't get much attention in our tradition. It makes a brief appearance in the book of Ecclesiastes and then is rarely heard from again.

This older, cyclic worldview probably reflected a more feminine way of thinking. Women tend to be lunar, men solar. They have cycles, men don't. Masculinity has a plan. It's about progress. Femininity—bound more closely to the generative cycle—tends to have its doubts.

Another Dimension of Time

In this older view of the world, time itself consists of a series of moments, going nowhere in particular, strung together like beads on a string. Most often you never notice them. But if you practice giving them your full attention, you realize they're always there. Without your noticing it, your whole life has been a series of them.

Sexual arousal, if you let it happen the way it's intended to, is all about revealing these moments. In fact, arousal is *designed* to keep you in the moment. That's what it *does*.

From the first day as a teenager that you get so aroused in someone's arms that you lose all track of time and suddenly it's 2:00 A.M. and your parents are frantic wondering where you are, to the day before your youngest child's wedding when you go to bed early to hold each other and maybe make love because the moments all seem to be flying by so fast, sexual arousal opens you up to another dimension of time.

Sex, as I'm forever telling patients in my office, is fundamentally a passive thing. The secret to good sex in a lasting relationship is to sanctify the erotic moment by paying attention to it in all its variety, without judgment.

Sometimes you will feel highly aroused, and sometimes it will be no more than a still, small voice. Part of being a sexual adult is learning to listen to that still, small voice.

That takes a bit of discipline. But the sexual self is thoroughly immature and quite incapable of discipline. So you have to parent your sexual self, using the same tools that good parents employ in guiding their children: gentleness, patience, and faith.

A good parent makes sure their child has a safe passage through childhood to adulthood. When you're a good parent to your sexual self, you ensure its safe passage through adulthood to a serene old age.

Faith is something that gets passed down from one generation to the next. The faith you learned as a child traveled a long way to reach you. Now it's your turn to pass it on to the next generation.

You may be just this year's flowers. But next year's flowers may bloom more brightly because you were here.

After the Rain

> To go to a funeral is to have sex afterward, if you can. Sex in marriage is the darkest and the best, a celebration of life's most capricious glory and its more permanent sorrow, when one faces separation from existence itself.
> —AVODAH OFFIT, *THE SEXUAL SELF*

My office buzzer rings. It's Emily, here for her three thirty appointment. I haven't seen her in a few weeks.

"It's really warm for November," she says. "Let's go outside."

I'm already comfortable and have no wish to go outside.

She gives me a pleading look. I get my coat.

It rained overnight, and now there are wet, yellow leaves all the way up and down the avenue. We cross at the traffic light and head into the trees.

There aren't many tourists in Strawberry Fields this time of year, and the street musicians have packed up their guitars until next spring. We find a nice dry bench overlooking the lake, which is still and gray under a warm gray sky.

Emily reaches inside her purse for a tissue.

"My father had to go back in the hospital again," she says.

"I'm sorry to hear that."

"No, it was okay—just for a few days, so they could adjust his pacemaker settings and some other stuff."

She looks out at the water.

"One day I came to visit him, and my mother was there already. They'd been kissing together or something. I think I surprised them. They both looked a little embarrassed."

She puts her hands in her coat pockets. "Strange to think of your parents sharing that kind of intimacy," she says.

Then Emily remembers something. She reaches in her bag and shows me a paperback copy of Avodah Offit's *The Sexual Self*.

"Where'd you get the book?" I ask.

"You mentioned it a long time ago," she says. "I found a used copy on Amazon."

Emily leafs through the book, looking for something.

"What's this mean?" she asks, and reads aloud:

"*To go to a funeral is to have sex afterward, if you can. Sex in marriage is the darkest and the best, a celebration of life's most capricious glory and its more permanent sorrow, when one faces separation from existence itself.*"

"I understand 'permanent sorrow,'" she says. "That's pretty obvious. But what's 'capricious glory'?"

I think for a moment, wondering how to put my thoughts into words.

"You know how most couples remember the first time they ever had sex?" I ask. "Well, when you and Sam are having sex, did you ever think about the fact that someday there'll be a *last* time?"

"No, I've never thought about that."

"I imagine your parents have thought about it. I think that's what Offit meant by 'capricious glory.' A joy in the moment, even though you don't know for sure how many moments like that you might have left."

"That sounds impossibly sad."

"Not if you've loved each other well. In some mystical way, love and sex are always about the future. In the erotic moment there's a feeling that says, '*Of course* there's a future for us. How could there not be, when we've loved each other so well?'"

"You know that makes no logical sense, right?"

"It's an act of faith. Love survives death."

"Is that what you believe?"

"As a therapist, I'd say it's an infantile wish. But I believe it with all my heart."

"Why?"

"Early imprinting, I guess. Your mother loves you, so you imagine the world must love you too."

"Even when you discover the rest of the world doesn't really love you?"

"Deep down, you still think that it must. As long as there's one person who loves you, you can't imagine the universe would ever just let you go."

Love and Attachment

The touch of mother's arms, breasts, and body had to be an early ecstasy for which we search again. Were it not for custom, most of us would stay close to our mother's bodies until we found some warm replacement. As it is, we are laid crying to rest by ourselves, left to learn very slowly that being alone is not a death.

—AVODAH OFFIT, *THE SEXUAL SELF*

"How are things with Sam?" I ask. "Still having good sex?"

"Sure," she says, putting her hands in the pockets of her coat. "But you know the two of us still don't really have much in common. It gets lonely sometimes."

Emily looks out at the water again. "It's probably just me," she says.

"You always *were* pretty solitary," I say.

"Yeah, why am I like that?" she asks.

"Some people just seem to have a knack for being alone. There's a classic psychology experiment from the 1960s—they'd take a child, one to two years old, playing in a room with its mother. On cue, Mom leaves suddenly, and the child gets upset. Then Mom comes back after three minutes, and they watch what the child does."

"That's awful. What's the point?"

"To see how they go about reattaching. Some kids get clingy and won't let Mom out of their sight for a long time. Some are upset for a few seconds, then they're fine. But there's a third group who look *superficially* like they're fine, but if you watch closely you see they're very stressed. They just handle it by shutting down."

"Maybe they're the ones with cold mothers?"

"It's not that simple. Some kids seem to have an innate capacity to say, *'The heck with this. From now on, I'm taking care of myself.'*"

"I can't believe they just shut down like that."

"The first researchers who noticed it were pretty surprised too.

They called it 'avoidance.' It's not as dramatic as when a child clings and cries and won't let go. If you're not tuned in you can easily miss it. But it's there."

"What happens to those kids? The ones who just shut down?"

"I'm sure there are lots of different possibilities. But if you look at the adults you know, some of them seem to have that quality. They're self-sufficient. They travel light, because they're not burdened by a lot of attachments."

"I think I have some of that."

"A lot of people do."

"Is that okay?"

"It has its advantages. But it's often originally a response to pain." Emily thinks for a moment.

"You think my mother abandoned me?"

"It doesn't have to be that dramatic. It could have been anything. Maybe something about her that confused you. Or something about *you* that confused *her*. Something neither of you knew quite what to do with. So you disconnected."

"I can see how that might have happened," she says.

Emily turns herself around to face me on the bench.

"I think this might be my last session," she says.

This feels abrupt, and a little shocking. I wonder what's going on. Is she just shutting down, like one of those kids in the attachment experiments?

"Was it something I said?" I ask.

"No. I'd been planning to tell you. I think I can handle it from here on out," she says.

Emily puts the book back in her bag. "I really want to thank you for teaching Sam and me how to have sex again," she says, standing up and brushing dust from her skirt.

"Hey, it's what I do," I say. "Are you still Two-Stepping?"

"Yup. Every time."

"Good. A lot of couples forget to do that."

She thanks me again, and we shake hands.

As she turns and heads up the West Drive toward the Great Lawn, I'm aware of a cold, tired feeling that I know is a kind of grief. Maybe it's the way she suddenly announced she wasn't coming back. Whatever happened long ago to Emily that launched her on her rather solitary path, maybe she's just given me a taste of it.

I hope Emily decides to tell Sam she's been feeling lonely. I'm sure he'd want to know that.

I'm glad they're still having good sex. Even people with strong avoidance traits need to regress to an infantile state once in a while with someone they care about.

I walk uphill back to Strawberry Fields, where it's already starting to get dark. By the time I get to Central Park West, it's nearly rush hour and the traffic has picked up. I grab a quick cup of coffee at a nearby convenience store, then head back to the office to see my last few patients of the evening.

A Wish

At 9:00 P.M., I lock up my office for the night. I look across the avenue to the park—now dark and forbidding on this moonless night.

Turning away from the park, I head west on Seventy-Second Street, then turn to walk downtown on Columbus Avenue. The stores are mostly closed, but the restaurants are brightly lit and full of people. A few places already have holiday lights up.

Above the street level are the windows of people's apartments. Having spent all day listening to people's stories, I can't help wondering about all the stories taking place above me tonight as I walk downtown.

Thirty-five years ago, Avodah Offit used to look out her terrace and wonder the same thing. On one occasion she thought to record the moment:

The windows across the courtyard are glowing. Behind them, people are watering plants, baking bread, fixing radiators, flipping television channels. Other windows are curtained, and beyond them, people might even be making love. Good for them. I wish them well. It's not easy to be successfully sexual these days, and perhaps it never was. I do what I can to help.

Now a third of a century later, the city is still an intimate place. Behind the windows above me on Columbus Avenue, people are having late dinners, reading, watching TV. I know from my office these days that not many New Yorkers have sex on weeknights. Mostly they're too tired.

But I imagine somewhere in one of the darkened windows there's a couple who are still in their first throes of passion on this weeknight at 9:00 P.M. I imagine they'll stay up most of the night, lost in each other's presence and wondering if this might be for real.

It's entirely possible this couple will never need my help. But while I have them in mind, I silently make them the following wish:

> *Pay attention to this moment. It won't come again. Moments like these have their mission, which is to inspire you to love. Love each other deeply and well.*
>
> *Be patient and kind to each other. In the place where you came together just now, you were as honest as small children, and just as vulnerable.*
>
> *The small children of your inner hearts will show you the way to heaven, if you let them. Let them run all the way up to heaven together, holding hands.*

Eleven Classic Sex-Knots, and How to Untie Them

Masters and Johnson famously referred to sexual response as a "natural function." You don't need to be taught to do it. Your body already knows how. You just need to get out of its way.

Unfortunately most of us have trouble staying out of our own way. When our bodies don't respond sexually as we'd like them to, we tend to react in ways that make matters worse. In Chapters 9 through 11 we referred to these kinds of situations as "sex-knots," and we discussed how to identify and untie several of the more classic ones.

As promised, here are the solutions to several more. I've arranged them roughly in order from most simple to most complex.

1

You don't feel anything during sex.

You think, "There must be something wrong with me."

This makes you lose all arousal.

Now you're *sure* there's something wrong with you.

If you don't feel anything during sex, that usually just means your sexual self isn't happy.

Your sexual self usually knows what it's doing. Maybe it's trying to tell you something.

Ask yourself: Was there a moment back there when you actually did feel something?

Good. See if you can "hit rewind." Go back there.

Once you're feeling something again, hold on to it and don't let it get away.

～～

It's normal to lose arousal in the presence of extreme negative thinking. As I mentioned in Chapter 5, we mental health folks have lots of ways to help people cope with so-called Automatic Negative Thoughts (ANTs). But most of these ways take more time and energy than is really practical while you're having sex.

During sex, it's usually best to just realize that it's an ANT and not give it any of your emotional energy. As the Buddhist sage Shunryu Suzuki taught, "Leave your front door and back door open. Let thoughts come and go. Just don't serve them tea."

Arousal that's been lost can almost always be regained. But that's much less likely to happen if you're freaking out.

ANTs only tend to hang around if you pay lots of attention to them. Don't serve them any tea, and they'll eventually get bored and go somewhere else.

Save your tea for after the ANTs have left. Then pour and enjoy.

2

There's no passion in your lovemaking.

You think, "This is never going to work."

Your partner thinks, "Nothing I do works."

Now there's even less passion.

You see the problem here, right?

It's that one word: *work*.

If you're *working* during sex, you're definitely doing it wrong.

Work tends to have a goal—and your sexual self just doesn't understand goals. Whether your goal is to impress your partner, give them an orgasm, get pregnant, make someone fall in love with you, or something else, attaching a goal to sex always carries some risk.

Your sexual self experiences the world very differently from you. For instance, you might imagine that a romantic weekend at a bed-and-breakfast resort would be just the thing to inspire passion. But your sexual self might just see it as more pressure to perform. I usually tell couples to nurture their erotic connection at home first, *before* heading out to the bed-and-breakfast.

A good first move is to learn the Two-Step (Chapter 6)—which is the world's easiest sex practice. It starts with just hanging out together in bed doing nothing at all, then letting your senses lead the way from there.

Sometimes a Two-Step might lead to a passionate encounter and sometimes not. But at least it starts you off from a place of honesty and acceptance—which, trust me, is the very best place to begin.

Do that every week for a month or two, and you may even begin to feel some passion again. *Then* go enjoy a weekend at the bed-and-breakfast.

You'll get more for your money.

3

Mary takes a long time to reach orgasm.

This worries her so much that she can't reach orgasm.

Why in the world would someone worry about how long it takes to reach orgasm?

I mean, what's the big deal? If it takes a long time, then it takes a long time.

The key thing is that it should be an *exciting* time!

As we discussed in Chapter 6, orgasm should be like dessert—a great end to a great meal. The best way to ensure a wonderful dessert experience is to make sure you've thoroughly enjoyed every course leading up to it.

Just make sure you're authentically aroused—you know, really dumb and happy.

Some people forget to make sure they stay aroused. They work so hard to get a climax that the longer it takes, the less and less aroused they feel.

If it's truly a challenge for Mary to reach orgasm—even when she's by herself, and even if she's highly turned on—then she might want to invest in a good vibrator, learn how to use it by herself, then experiment with using it with a partner.

After all, life is difficult. Sex should be easy.

An orgasm is just a reflex, really—as we discussed in Chapter 2. Best not to get too emotional about a reflex.

Save your emotions for more important stuff.

4

Jim feels frustrated when he can't bring Mary to orgasm.

Mary feels his frustration.

This makes it even more difficult for Mary to reach orgasm.

The idea that it's one person's responsibility to give another person an orgasm can be the source of all kinds of trouble. Both giver and receiver can easily feel under too much pressure to make it happen.

Jim may be intensely attracted to Mary, but if he ends up stroking Mary's vulva for half an hour hoping to bring her to orgasm, by the end of that time he may no longer feel so turned on. She'll quickly realize there's no passion in it—which obviously won't be much of an aphrodisiac for her.

The alternative, which I highly recommend, is that Jim's primary attention should be to *his own* arousal. Then Mary can just enjoy *her* own arousal with a clear conscience.

You don't have to have a PhD to know that's going to make it easier for her to come.

If there's something special that Mary needs from Jim in order to orgasm—a special kind of stroking, or thrusting, or whatever—then by all means she should ask for that.

But whatever it is Mary needs from him, Jim should take responsibility for making sure he can sustain it without losing his own arousal.

Some men try to get all creative, trying to find new and interesting kinds of stimulation for their female partners. That's okay as long as it's fun for both of you. But it's often a better idea for a man to consider himself simply the rhythm section of the orchestra.

Just give her a steady beat to work with, then sit back and let her riff on it all she wants.

5

Jim doesn't really like to do cunnilingus.

He does it with Mary because he knows it's the best way for her to reach orgasm.

But she can't reach orgasm because she knows he doesn't really like it.

Many people think the purpose of oral sex is to stimulate your partner to orgasm. Not so.

The purpose of oral sex is to turn yourself on.

As I mentioned in Chapter 5, you shouldn't feel you're "giving" someone oral sex.

Better to think of it as "taking."

If your partner gets so excited by your mouth on their penis or vulva that they have an orgasm—hey, that's a plus. But don't make it the primary purpose.

I know this is different from what it says in the other sex books. But trust me. If you consistently do something for your partner that doesn't really turn you on, eventually it will sap your erotic energy. In the long run, that won't be so great for your partner either.

For some people, oral sex is somewhat of an acquired taste. Others never really get to liking it—even with a partner who turns them on in every other way.

Society has a bit of a double standard when it comes to this. Some women just love having their partner's penis in their mouth, and others don't. Everyone in the civilized world knows you should never pressure a woman to take your penis in her mouth if she doesn't really enjoy it.

Best to treat cunnilingus the same way. If, for whatever reason, your partner doesn't enjoy doing it, then go figure out some other way for them to enjoy your vulva that turns *both* of you on.

For instance, let's say cunnilingus has always been Mary's favorite kind of lovemaking with other partners. But it's never been especially Jim's thing.

In a perfect world, you'd fill out a questionnaire about this on a first date. But by the time many couples get around to sharing this information with each other, they're already deeply in love.

What to do?

Well, for starters, Jim and Mary might get more curious about each other's experiences in bed.

What exactly doesn't Jim like about cunnilingus? Is it Mary's scent? Does he feel claustrophobic with his head between her legs? Does he feel somehow "unmanly" in that position?

The answers to these questions might suggest all sorts of creative solutions.

What exactly does Mary like so much about cunnilingus? His warm breath on her clitoris? The texture of his tongue? His total attention to her vulva?

Assume you haven't exhausted all the options in the world for getting these things.

6

Mark has sex with Jenny and can't get hard.

Jenny gets very upset with him.

Now he *really* can't get hard.

The conventional script says a man should always be hard in bed. The truth is, men tend to get erections when they're happy and lose them when they're unhappy.

Unfortunately, losing an erection is right at the top of the list of things that can make a man unhappy—so the whole thing can easily snowball.

A woman will sometimes get upset when her man can't get an erection because she thinks this means he's not attracted to her. But that's rarely the case. Usually it's that he's upset about something.

Whatever is making him unhappy, it's not going to be helped by throwing a lot of emotion at it. Instead, it's usually best to treat the whole thing as matter-of-factly as possible.

Mark should try not to apologize for his lack of an erection. Instead, he might ask Jenny if she'd let him enjoy her body for his own pleasure—with the understanding that he probably won't get hard yet since the conditions aren't yet right.

Jenny might tell Mark that she's sorry she freaked out on him, but that it's really important for her to know she turns him on. So if he wants to show her some passionate attention, she'd welcome that. But no intercourse for now, since it's clear he's not ready for that yet.

You'd be surprised how many guys will get hard, once there's no pressure to do so.

Many men have *physical* problems with their erections—not just psychological ones. This is particularly common in older men, but it occurs in many younger men as well. In such cases, any of the so-called PDE5 inhibitor medications (Viagra, Cialis, et cetera) can be a gift from God.

Many women feel personally insulted if their male partners have to use medication to get hard. But this makes as much sense as a man getting insulted because his wife needs a lubricant to get sufficiently wet.

Sure, it's a great ego boost if your partner gets and stays hard or wet without assistance. But remember what we said above about goals during sex. If you make your partner's hardness or wetness into a goal, there's a good chance it won't work.

Don't focus so much on your partner's arousal. Just take care of your own. In general that's going to be much more erotic.

7

Mark has sex with Jenny and can't get hard.

She's very nice about it, but he still feels humiliated.

Mark spends all the next day masturbating to prove he can still get hard.

By the end of the day, he's even having trouble getting hard by himself.

Clearly part of the problem is that Mark's penis is exhausted. But there's also the fact that he's been masturbating with a specific and not very erotic goal in mind: to reassure himself that he's okay.

When a man has been unable to get hard in the presence of a much-desired partner, he'll ordinarily be vulnerable to negative *obsessions* about himself—unwanted thoughts like "I'm impotent" or "I'm not a real man." Compulsively masturbating will give him momentary relief from these obsessions.

The problem is that compulsions only reduce obsessions momentarily. Shortly afterward, Mark's obsessions will come back even stronger. Which will put him under even more pressure to keep masturbating.

Eventually both self-stimulation and partner sex will become entirely compulsive, and Mark will lose all awareness of whether he's feeling excited or not.

At some point his sexual self will likely call a stop to this nonsense by shutting down completely. Which will most likely throw him into outright panic.

The best thing Mark can do now if he wants to prevent this from happening is to stop masturbating for a while, until he calms down enough to distinguish whether he's genuinely excited or not. Then he should only masturbate if he feels excited—not just to test his ability to get hard, or to quiet an obsessive worry.

The next time Mark sees Jenny, he might to want to use some of the suggestions from Chapter 3—such as avoiding intercourse until he gets to know her a little better.

Many men who experience this particular sex-knot are so distressed that it's an act of mercy to write them a prescription for Viagra or Cialis. In the long run, sex therapy would probably be a better idea. But sex therapy requires a committed couple, and Mark and Jenny aren't a committed couple yet.

Under the circumstances, Cialis can be like a set of training wheels—useful for building your confidence again until you've stopped panicking and are ready to take them off.

8

The next time Mark spends the night with Jenny, he gets hard but worries it won't last.

So he tries to penetrate as quickly as possible.

In the process, he loses his erection.

Your sexual self has no idea why anyone would ever want to hurry anything. Force it to hurry, and it may get upset and quit on you.

Remember the 0 to 100 arousal scale we talked about in Chapter 9? If Mark is like most young men, he'll only need about a 20 of arousal to get hard. And when he gets to a 20 he'll want to penetrate right away.

But that's a mistake. Better to wait until he gets to a 40—not just hard but fully aroused. Then he'll have arousal to spare. Even if he loses a bit of it while trying to penetrate, or while putting on a condom, he'll still be hard.

Which will make him happy. Which means he'll stay hard. And so on and so on.

It's a leap of faith to wait until you're fully aroused before penetrating, but it's well worth it.

By the way, during intercourse many men think they have to keep thrusting to stay hard. Which of course is ridiculous.

I always ask the men in my office, "Did you need a lot of physical stimulation to get hard during foreplay?"

The answer is usually no. During foreplay, the sight and feel of a partner's body is ordinarily quite enough to give a man an erection.

But men tend to forget this during intercourse. They forget that the same person that attracted them during foreplay is still very much there, eager to be enjoyed.

Motionless intercourse can be the best intercourse of all—once you realize that even during intercourse there can be lots of other sources of eroticism besides genital-genital rubbing.

"Yeah," say the men in my office after I explain this to them. "That makes sense."

I've yet to figure out why the idea doesn't occur to them on their own.

Thrusting can feel wonderful, of course. Just don't make it compulsive.

Remember to stop and smell the roses every once in a while.

9

Bonnie has no desire for sex.

Every time Bonnie shows Pat affection, Pat ends up wanting sex.

Bonnie withdraws.

Pat feels unloved.

Seeking reassurance, Pat pressures Bonnie for sex.

Bonnie thinks, "Pat doesn't love me anymore. All Pat wants is sex."

Bonnie feels unloved.

Now Bonnie has *absolutely* no desire for sex.

We don't know what happened to make Bonnie lost desire in the first place. But by this point Bonnie and Pat are so sex-knotted that it almost doesn't matter. As long as Pat keeps pressuring Bonnie for sex, and as long as Bonnie keeps withdrawing, they're going to stay stuck this way forever.

The first step in unraveling this particular sex-knot is for Bonnie to explain to Pat that when she feels pressured to have sex, this makes her feel unloved. Pat will almost certainly reply that Bonnie's refusing sex makes *Pat* feel unloved.

Bonnie and Pat can then talk together about what they each need in order to feel loved.

Maybe Pat is someone who needs to feel loved through physical intimacy. Maybe Bonnie needs long, heartfelt conversations in order to feel loved. Maybe Pat isn't very good at heartfelt conversations.

I tell couples it's normal to have conflicts of this sort. The question is, what are you going to do about them?

If Pat needs sex in order to feel loved, then Bonnie might wonder: Exactly how much sex does Pat need, and what kind?

Does Pat always need an orgasm? If so, then maybe some "lazy sex" once in a while (Chapter 9) might help bridge the disparity between their levels of desire. If not, then some regular "simmering" (Chapter 5) might go a long way.

If Bonnie needs heartfelt conversation in order to feel loved, then Pat might wonder: Would Bonnie be more open to erotic closeness if it's preceded by fifteen minutes of Pat actively listening to what Bonnie has to say? Active listening is a skill that can be taught, and Pat might be motivated to learn it—especially if this might result in Pat getting more sex.

People often lose desire when they feel a situation is hopeless—or when they feel helpless to change it. Once in a while someone in Bonnie's position may even rediscover an interest in sex, once they start to feel more empowered.

Sometimes the best aphrodisiac is to regain some sense of hope.

10

Bonnie says no to sex.

This makes Pat feel needy.

Pat's neediness is a big turnoff for Bonnie.

Bonnie keeps saying no to sex.

Feeling needy in a relationship usually means you don't have enough power.

The only good solution is to get more power.

I don't mean dominance. (Though there's nothing wrong with dominance, if that's what gets the two of you going.) I mean the power that comes from taking care of your own emotional needs.

Pat has to find a way to take better care of his or her own emotional needs. Then Pat can approach Bonnie from a position of strength. In Chapter 12 we called this "standing your ground."

"Look," Pat might say to Bonnie. "I realize I've been wrong—expecting you to provide sex like it was some kind of emotional first aid. I can see how that might have turned you off."

Note that Pat isn't apologizing, or looking for forgiveness or reassurance. Pat is just stating the facts—without a whole lot of emotion. That's a more powerful position.

Bonnie might be a little thrown off balance by this.

"How do I know you won't go back to being needy and insecure tomorrow?" she might say.

"All I can do is tell you what I know right now," Pat might answer, staying in charge of his or her own emotions.

Hmm, Bonnie might think. *Maybe this isn't as hopeless as I thought.*

The sexual self is naturally attracted to power. And the most powerful thing you can do in an intimate encounter is to take full responsibility for yourself and give the other person the freedom to do the same.

11

Hank doesn't initiate sex.

Jamie gets angry because Hank doesn't initiate sex.

When Jamie gets angry, Hank doesn't feel like initiating sex.

There are many people whose primary erotic orientation is to be the object of desire. This kind of orientation is very common in straight women, as we discussed in Chapter 7. Some gay men and lesbians are oriented this way too.

When someone whose primary erotic orientation is to be the object of desire finds themselves in a relationship where they don't feel desired, this will often feel like a crisis.

Let's assume that Jamie's primary motivation for sex is to feel desired. Jamie might enjoy initiating sex once in awhile for fun. But if Hank completely stops initiating sex and Jamie has to initiate on a regular basis, Jamie will eventually get angry.

Why would Hank stop initiating sex? We don't know. It could be something simple, like the fact that for one reason or another sex with Jamie was unsatisfying. Or maybe the sex was fine, and the problem was something deeper and more emotional.

The more Jamie gets upset that Hank won't initiate, the more hopeless Hank will feel about ever being able to please Jamie. Which on the face of it makes no sense at all. The only reason Jamie got angry in the first place is because Hank wouldn't initiate sex. Why doesn't Hank just initiate?

Sometimes there are deep emotional reasons. Often someone like Hank turns out to be reenacting something from his childhood involving a harsh, critical parent. See our discussion of enactments in Chapter 17.

Very often it turns out that the person in Jamie's position is reenacting something from his or her childhood as well—perhaps *identifying* with a harsh, critical parent, as we saw in Chapter 14.

Sometimes it's useful to wonder why someone like Jamie chose someone like Hank to begin with. Perhaps Hank has other good qualities that more than compensate for his relative passivity.

Sex-knots involving initiation (or the lack of it) are the most likely to require professional help to unravel. Hank will need to learn better leadership skills, and he'll need to learn to use power wisely in a relationship. In addition, Hank and Jamie will each need to learn to calmly "stand their ground" with each other, instead of just getting angry or withdrawing.

In the meantime, it's important that they keep having sex. I usually recommend that deeply sex-knotted couples like Hank and Jamie learn to Two-Step (Chapter 15), since this is something a couple can do in a wider range of emotional circumstances than might be possible with conventional lovemaking.

Good Two-Stepping can help a couple like Hank and Jamie stay calm enough to risk becoming emotionally connected again—even if they're otherwise completely frustrated with each other.

With any luck, it might also make them feel more like allies than adversaries.

Sometimes that can be the most important thing of all.

Notes

v. *"We are like islands in the sea . . ."* This is the version that's conventionally quoted. But if William James ever uttered these exact words, they do not appear ever to have been published as such.

In "Essays in Psychical Research," published in *American Magazine* in October 1909, James wrote the following: *"Out of my experience, such as it is (and it is limited enough) one fixed conclusion dogmatically emerges, and that is this, that we with our lives are like islands in the sea, or like trees in the forest. The maple and the pine may whisper to each other with their leaves. . . . But the trees also commingle their roots in the darkness underground, and the islands also hang together through the ocean's bottom. Just so there is a continuum of cosmic consciousness, against which our individuality builds but accidental fences, and into which our several minds plunge as into a mother-sea or reservoir."*

PART I: YOUR SEXUAL SELF

Chapter 1: Rules of the Heart

9 *Since 1978, when AASECT prohibited nudity and physical touch in the office . . .* American Association of Sex Educators, Counselors, and Therapists (1978).

12 *Masters and Johnson* For a highly readable account of Masters and Johnson's original experiments at Washington University in the 1950s and '60s, see Maier (2009, pp. 95–115).

12 *Psychological Aspects of Arousal* In "Three Dimensions of Depth of Involvement in Human Sexual Response," Donald Mosher argues that sexual arousal can be thought of as like a hypnotic trance. The most intense and meaningful sexual experiences tend to be the deepest trances, where you feel most profoundly absorbed. See also Klein and Robbins (1998, pp. 144–47). I agree, but I think we can go further and say that sexual trance states (and possibly hypnotic trances as well) represent *regressions* to more infantile states of mind, as we'll discuss in Chapter 3.

Mosher describes three dimensions of sexual arousal—"sexual trance," "partner engagement," and "role enactment." My own notion of "sex of the heart" doesn't fit exactly with any of his categories—but I believe it would fit closest to the first, with a bit of the second thrown in. I agree with Mosher that the best sex might include a generous helping of all three.

14 "*the trouble with most books on sex . . .*" Paul Joannides, personal communication.

Chapter 2: The Sexual Self in Action

15 *Go to your bosom.* Shakespeare, *Measure for Measure*, Act II, Scene 2.

16 Many parts of Offit's *The Sexual Self* are now fairly out of date. Her next book, *Night Thoughts* (1981), a series of essays on various topics in clinical sexuality, has held up better and is probably a better place to start for a modern reader wishing to sample her writing.

19 *staying on the couch* Helen Kaplan may have originated this technique. She was famous for telling couples to stay on the couch.

22 *American Psychiatric Association.* See Drescher (2015) and Drescher and Merlino (2007).

23 *Ordeals like the kind Sarina went through* Dozens of nations around the world still regard same-sex sexual acts as criminal, and there are many places where sex between two men is still punishable by death (Nichols 2013, p. 23).

23 *a catalog of all our diversity* See Nichols (2014, pp. 317–19).

24 *"mostly straight" or "heteroflexible"* See Savin-Williams (2016).

Chapter 3: Be my Baby

25 *"We live to be touched."* Offit (1983, p. 20).

25 *"It was a hot and humid August day . . ."* Whoever wrote the piece from which this quotation is taken apparently never published it themselves. The earliest version that I know of—somewhat different from the one I've included in Chapter 3—appears in Kahn (1989, p. 54), where it's stated that the author is unknown. A version nearly identical to Kahn's is used as part of the Our Whole Lives sexuality education curriculum of the Unitarian Universalist Association—again without attribution.

The piece I've quoted in Chapter 3 is very similar in style and subject matter to the prose poem at the start of Alayne Yates' book, *Sex Without Shame* (Yates 1978, p. 11)—which leads me to suspect that Yates may be the author of the piece in question. But I have been unable to confirm this.

26 *mother-infant bonding* The *Three Essays on the Theory of Sexuality* (1905) was Freud's original and most complete statement of his idea that the physical gratifications of early childhood might have something to do with adult erotic experience. Freud thought adult sexual hunger and the infant's urge to breastfeed were both emanations of a kind of bioenergetic "drive."

Most modern writers have long since given up on Freud's drive theory. But there is still a broad consensus that the experiences of infancy and early childhood help form the template for adult sexuality (Dinnerstein, 1976 Yates, 1978 Scharff, 1982 Scharff and Scharff 1991; Zolbrod, 2005 Johnson 2008, 2013), and that adult erotic experience reevokes aspects of infantile life.

For example, Dorothy Dinnerstein writes that sex "*resonates, more literally than any other part of our experience, with the massive orienting passions that first take shape in pre-verbal, pre-rational human infancy*" (1976, p. 15). While this idea is not testable in a scientific sense, I can't imagine working as a sex therapist without it.

29 *survivors of sexual abuse* See Haines (2007) and Maltz (2012) for more detailed information regarding the effects of sexual betrayal and abuse on the sexual self. See also Jack Morin's *The Erotic Mind*—especially Section II, "Troublesome Turn-Ons" (1995, pp. 169–262). Sexual abuse of boys and young men is less often discussed, but is also extremely common (Gartner, 1999, 2005).

34 *'shy penis'* Simply imposing a "ban on intercourse" can resolve many cases of psychogenic ED, as we'll discuss further at the end of Chapter 9.

Chapter 4: Selfishly Yours

37 *"Being chosen by the one you chose is one of the glories of falling in love . . ."* Perel (2006, p. 20).

37 *"I am my beloved's, and my beloved is mine."* Song of Songs 6:3.

37 *our possessive instincts* The tension between our generous and possessive instincts has been resolved in different ways by various cultures. In *Sex at Dawn* (2010), Christopher Ryan and Cacilda Jetha argue that preagricultural human societies were nomadic and cooperative and therefore put a high value on generosity—often even sharing sex partners. The invention of agriculture ten thousand years ago may have put the notion of "mine" front and center—*my* land, *my* tools, *my* spouse. Since then, it probably wasn't much of a stretch to feel you owned exclusive sexual rights to your partner's body. See Notes for Chapter 15.

38 *healthy narcissism* In his 1914 paper, *On Narcissism: An Introduction,* Freud identified healthy narcissism as part of the universal instinct for self-preservation. Meana (2010, p. 113) reviews recent research suggesting that nonpathological narcissism may be fundamental for sexual enjoyment.

38 *the essence of growing up* As Dinnerstein writes (1976, p. 60), *"The fact that human infants receive such nearly perfect care seduces them into fantasies which are inevitably crushed, fantasies of a world that automatically obeys, even anticipates, their wishes. The loss of this infantile illusion of omnipotence . . . is an original and basic human grief."*

Unfortunately many children's early environments are such that infantile illusions of omnipotence quickly give way to feelings of powerlessness and hopelessness. Many children learn to adapt by denying their right to independent pleasure (Bader, 2002, pp. 17–24). See Notes to Chapter 17.

42 *at the court of a powerful rajah* Friday (1973, pp. 37–39).

47 *Shame makes you want to run and hide . . .* Shame researcher Brené Brown (2007, p. 5) writes, "Shame is the intensely painful feeling or experience of believing we are flawed and therefore unworthy of acceptance and belonging." Group membership was essential for survival early in human history (and is only somewhat less essential now). I imagine humans originally developed the capacity to feel shame because shame was useful in enforcing standards for group behavior.

As Brown (2007, 2010) notes, shame *disconnects* us from others. Arousal, on the other hand, evokes early feelings of deep connection. So it's not surprising that shame and arousal are often mutually exclusive. (See Bader 2002, p. 81.)

Chapter 5: The Art of the Easy

49 *"Life is difficult."* This first line of M. Scott Peck's *The Road Less Traveled* (1978) is an adaptation of the first of the Buddha's Four Noble Truths: "Life is suffering."

49 *"It's natural for humans to seek out joy . . ."* Northrup (2010, p. 250).

50 *"Does fingering even work???"* Wendy Strgar's October 11, 2013 article, "Foreplay's Harvest," is viewable at https://makinglovesustainable.com/foreplays-harvest/

50 *She Comes First* In Chapter 20 of *She Comes First*, Ian Kerner recommends that a man provide his female partner with "three assurances." The first of these is, *"Going down on her turns you on. You enjoy it as much as she does."* My experience in talking with many hundreds of men over the years is that there are some for whom this is true, and some for whom it just isn't—even after extensive counseling about the pleasures of cunnilingus.

52 *The New Sex Therapy* Kaplan (1974, pp. 121–36).

55 *Many sex books offer techniques on how to deal with ANTS in bed.* The so-called first wave of brief, practical psychotherapies were the behavioral therapies. These consisted essentially of doing things you were afraid to do, so that your mind would learn they weren't really dangerous. Masters and Johnson's original treatment techniques were part of this tradition—as were most of the recommended practices in California psychologist Bernie Zilbergeld's original *Male Sexuality* (first published in 1978).

The second wave of brief, practical therapies consisted of variations on so-called cognitive therapy, which recommended identifying automatic negative thoughts (ANTs) and consciously changing them into more positive ones. Zilbergeld's *The New Male Sexuality* (1992; revised 1999) featured a new chapter, "Getting Your Mind on Your Side," (pp. 263–74), with cognitive-style interventions to counter negative thinking.

Zilbergeld died in 2002, just before the arrival of a third wave—the *mindfulness-based* brief therapies. These third-wave therapies recommend that rather than trying to *change* negative thoughts, it's usually more effective just not to get too emotionally involved with them. Third-wave therapists highlight the importance of "metacognitive awareness," the ability to simply *observe* thoughts as mental events.

Chapter 6: Two Roads to Orgasm

61 "*. . . yes I said yes I will Yes.*" Joyce (1922). When Molly Bloom speaks this passage in *Ulysses*, it's likely she's saying "yes" to penis-in-vagina penetration rather than to orgasm. Reliable contraception was harder to find in Joyce's day, so penetration was a much bigger deal.

61 ... *orgasm should be like dessert.* .... Sex therapist Marty Klein, quoted in Harriet Lerner's *Marriage Rules* (2013, p. 121), makes much the same point.

64 *"girl-gasms"* Serano (2007, pp. 65–76). The quotations are from pages 69, 70, and 71. Serano rightly cautions against generalizing from one person's experience of hormone treatment, since others' experiences on hormones will no doubt be different. But I find her descriptions too interesting not to include them here.

Emily Nagoski refers to *"extended orgasms"* and includes a good recipe on p. 343 of *Come as You Are* (2015).

65 *"In a word, the female orgasm is 'yes.'"* Feeney (2014).

65 *sexual accelerators and sexual brakes* The technical name for this idea is "the dual control model" (Janssen and Bancroft 2007; Carpenter et al. 2008; Bancroft et al. 2009; Graham, Sanders, and Millhausen 2006). Nagoski's *Come as You Are* provides an excellent introduction to the dual control model (pp. 42–69), and includes relevant self-assessment scales for women.

65 *a flock of birds* Nagoski (2015, pp. 282–85).

66 *resources available online* www.omgyes.com has an extensive video reference collection where real women discuss (and demonstrate) the techniques they've found most helpful. And www.dodsonandross.com has an excellent video collection with clips for rental download illustrating masturbation techniques.

66 *her "inner clitoris"* For their landmark book *A New View of a Woman's Body*, the Federation of Feminist Women's Health Centers (1981, pp. 33–57) cataloged the parts of the inner and outer clitoris, giving some of them names for the first time. Chalker (2000) and Kerner (2004) discuss these parts in detail. Northrup (2010, p. 234) refers to the totality as "the clitoral system." Barmak (2016, p. 29), citing Jannini et al. (2014), refers to an overarching "clitourethrovaginal complex."

66 *vibrators* Selecting a vibrator can be a bit like choosing a vacuum cleaner. Power is important. Just as with vacuum cleaners, the plug-in ones have historically been able to deliver much more power. But new technologies have now allowed some of the larger, rechargeable battery-operated devices to catch up in this regard. Feel free to write me if you need specific recommendations.

67 *The Two-Step* I originally developed this technique—with the help of individuals and couples like Carmen and Scott—for low-desire couples who needed something to get them started on "sex-dates." There's a simple Two-Step recipe in Chapter 15 that can be modified any number of ways.

70 *"mindfulness"* I tend to recommend Jon Kabat-Zinn's *Mindfulness for Beginners* (2012). Its chapters are extremely short, which makes them easier to experience in the moment. For women, the last chapter of Nagoski's *Come as You Are* (2015, pp. 294–335) provides a useful orientation regarding mindfulness and nonjudgment.

70 *Mindfulness is just something that happens naturally . . .* This formulation is taken from Kabat-Zinn (2012, p. 17). "Mindfulness-Based Stress Reduction" (MBSR) courses are now available all over the world—just Google "MBSR" and your zip code—as well as online at the University of Massachusetts's Center for Mindfulness http://www.umassmed.edu /cfm/.

71 *Mindfulness-Based Sex Therapy (MBST)* As of this writing, Brotto's group-based Mindfulness-Based Sex Therapy (MBST) is only available at the University of British Columbia in Vancouver. MBST is adapted from Mindfulness-Based Cognitive Therapy for Depression (MBCT; Segal et al. 2013)—as is a protocol in development by Agnes Kocsis and John Newbury-Helps (2016)

called Mindfulness in Sex Therapy and Intimate Relationships (MSIR).

Since Lonnie Barbach (1975) began reporting on her success using support groups to help women who were having trouble reaching orgasm, many practitioners have noted that a special magic often happens when groups of women get together to talk about sex. Gina Ogden (2006, 2008) has developed group programs for women to explore mind-, body-, heart-, and spirit-aspects of their sexuality (www.4-dnetwork.com). Pamela Madsen (2011, 2016) holds "Back to the Body" retreats for women, combining individual sexological bodywork with intensive but fully-clothed group experiences (www.backtothebody.org). Nicole Daedone guides groups of women in a sex practice she calls Orgasmic Meditation (Daedone 2011, Snyder 2012). And writer Sarah Barmak describes a "female sexual underground" of women who gather to do group masturbation, to get aroused together in various other ways, and to share empowering information about sexuality that isn't easily found in mainstream culture (Barmak 2016, pp. 100–14). These mind-body practices hearken back to the early days of sex therapy, when sexual healing was seen as part of a broader humanistic enterprise (Tiefer, 2006).

71 *vulvar mindfulness* This is a modification of a technique mentioned in Julia Heiman and Joseph LoPiccolo's book, *Becoming Orgasmic* (1976). It generally begins with taking a bath or a shower, paying attention to all the sensations of being in the water, smelling the soap, seeing your skin, et cetera—then moves on to a visual mindfulness exercise where you use a handheld mirror to look at your vulva, paying attention to perceptions, thoughts, and feelings as you experience them. As with the more rigorous variants of sensate focus discussed in Chapter 16 (Weiner and Avery-Clark 2014, 2017), there is no pleasure goal per se (Brotto, 2016a).

72 *"peace at the center and core of the universe"* Nagoski (2015, p. 292).

73 *Female and male are neither opposites nor mutually exclusive.* See Serano (2007, p. 19).

PART II: WOMEN AND MEN

Chapter 7: The Woman in the Mirror

80 *"Erotic Self-Focus"* Meana and Fertel (2015), Fertel (2015). See also Bogaert and Brotto, "Object of Desire Self-Consciousness" (2014), and Ogas and Gaddam on "self-directed erotic cues" (2011, pp. 108–13).

Bogaert, Visser, and Pozzebon report that "object of desire self-consciousness" plays a prominent role in most women's sexual/romantic fantasies (Bogaert, Visser, and Pozzebon 2015). Jill Weber (2013, pp. 1–23) describes how some young women get trapped into a cycle of serial hookups in an attempt to "fix" feelings of low desirability.

84 *"Juego"* Perel (2010, p. 35).

84 *Is "Juego" just the human version of what female rats do?* Sexologist John Bancroft in *Human Sexuality and Its Problems* (2009, p. 132) asks, "Does the female rat enjoy the mounting and intromission, or is her reward the pacing and control of the male's behavior . . . ?" There's apparently some experimental evidence for the latter, and Bancroft wonders whether this may be somewhat true for many human females as well. Marta Meana notes that animal research "supports the rewarding nature of evoking desire in potential mates" (2010, p. 107).

86 *Everyone's wiring is different, so it's usually best to ask.* Glennon Doyle, in her recent memoir *Love Warrior* (2016, p. 238), recounts how being grabbed by her husband inevitably turns

her off. "I want to be invited to affection," she writes, "not ambushed by it." Every person's relationship to touch is distinctive and bears the imprint of both their natural "wiring" and their previous experiences in life.

86 *"And so I started hating my body . . ."* Doyle (2016, p. 187).

87 *". . . a cruel discovery for young girls . . ."* Foley, Kope, and Sugrue (2011, p. 22).

88 *. . . the conventional script has never had much to say about a woman's own sexual pleasure* The man-as-subject/woman-as-object aspect of the conventional script shows up in unexpected places. Jessica Benjamin (1988, p. 87) describes a newborn nursery where boy babies' bassinettes carry blue labels that say *"I'm a boy!"* while those with girl babies carry pink labels saying *"It's a girl."* As Benjamin writes, *"The infant girl was already presented to the world not as a potential 'I,' but as an object, 'It.'"*
   Dinnerstein (1976, pp. 105–112) sees in this *"woman as It"* phenomenon an infantile equation of mother with a kind of primordial substance—as in "mother earth," "mother nature," or even the *mater* in "material." According to Dinnerstein, mother is the "non-self" or "other" against which the self of the infant differentiates.

88 *Girls & Sex* Orenstein (2016, pp. 1–43).

88 *what to do when your partner catches you* Tolman (2002) and Orenstein (2016) note that many young women experience remarkably little direct pleasure from partner sex. Doyle (2016, pp. 20–21) describes her own experience of this in vivid detail.
   Tolman notes that adolescent girls typically don't discuss their own sexual desire unless specifically asked about it, and even then one often has to listen carefully to discern an authentic "erotic voice" (2002, pp. 25–26, 41). Tolman sees this as evidence that girls are under pressure in a patriarchal culture to discon-

nect from erotic feelings—and from their erotic bodies (ibid., p. 54). In fact, themes of connection (or reconnection) with the erotic body permeate the sex self-help literature for women (Ogden 2006, 2008; Daedone 2011; Madsen 2011, 2016).

As Tolman sees it, female autonomous desire inevitably leads to dilemmas of one kind or another, from the risk of early motherhood to the risk of a damaged reputation. Many women try to safely contain desire within stable conventional relationships (Tolman 2002, pp. 80–81)—but this works better for some women than for others. Claire Dederer's recent memoir, *Love and Trouble*, describes the author's difficulty corralling her desire within conventional bounds—both as an adolescent and later as a middle-aged woman (Dederer 2017). The book's title seems to affirm Tolman's thesis that in a patriarchal culture, a women's autonomous desire inherently poses a dilemma of some kind.

Tolman writes that in her research a subject's "erotic voice" is frequently accompanied by other internal voices *responding* to the presence of desire. These might include *anti*-erotic voices (Tolman 2002, pp. 210–14). Dederer, writing in *The Atlantic* (2014), says much the same thing—that her own experience of desire *"come with an endless internal monologue—or maybe dialogue, or maybe babel. My desire is always guessing, often second-guessing. Female lust is a powerful force, but it surges in the form of an interrogation, rather than a statement. Not I want this but Do I want this? What exactly do I want? How about now? And now?"*

88 *Society both idealizes and disparages women* . . . For additional commentary regarding the latter, see Serano (2007) and Valenti (2016).

Chapter 8: Men at Work

89 *"My husband and I met on a volleyball court . . ."* The opening quotation is from Pogrebin (2016), who notes, "I was not just

sunning by the pool watching my future husband play volley ball. I was across the net playing against him, albeit in the yellow bikini."

90 *... simple acts of thoughtfulness can count just as much as grand gestures.* This point is noted by John Gray in *Men Are from Mars, Women Are from Venus* (2012, p. 199).

90 *When the first conflict arises between your wife and your family of origin ...* As Gottman and Silver write in *The Seven Principles for Making Marriage Work,* "The only way out of this dilemma is for the husband to side with his wife against his mother" (2015, p. 202).

93 *"There was energy here, a power of some kind in the way he worked."* The quotation is from Waller (1992, p. 88).

In the scene from which this passage is taken, Iowa home-maker Francesca Johnson watches Waller's fictional *National Geographic* photographer Robert Kincaid set up a shoot, and becomes aware she's starting to lubricate. Several hours later, they're in each other's arms.

In the first few years after *The Bridges of Madison County* was published, *National Geographic* received thousands of letters asking for information about Kincaid. Many people found it difficult to accept the fact that he didn't exist (Lamb, 1995).

94 *"He just uses my body for his own pleasure ..."* I'm obviously not the first to wonder why submission and surrender often work as erotic fantasy. Perhaps it's a deep imprint from millennia past, when there were no institutions to prevent women being taken by force. The words "raped" and "ravished" originally had the same meaning. We are an undeniably violent species, and throughout human history women have been vulnerable to sexual assault.

Paradoxically, though, many women get turned on by fanta-sizing about scenes of submission and even helplessness that would be traumatic in reality—what Jessica Benjamin calls "the problem of domination" (Benjamin 1988). *Story of O*—in which a young woman voluntarily becomes a nameless, faceless sex slave—was written by a woman, for women's enjoyment (Réage, 1954; Benjamin, 1988, pp. 55–65). Even today dominant men still attract scores of women, while submissive ones often can't get a date.

Is a woman's fantasy of being overpowered by an aggressive, dominant partner a holdover from thousands of years ago when such a partner would have been her best guarantee of survival? Is it a kind of transgenerational Stockholm syndrome? Or is it, as Michael Bader (2002) suggests, a roundabout way of overcoming internal obstacles to pleasure and safety? One colleague tells me it's the only way she can shut off her mind. Whatever the reason, this part of the conventional script still exerts a powerful influence on mating in our time.

95 *"Most of us get turned on at night by the very things that we'll demonstrate against during the day."* Quoted in Gottlieb (2014).

96 *If the father is domineering, the son becomes as un-domineering as he can.* Bader (2009, pp. 27–37) theorizes that many men feel uncomfortable acting more "passionately ruthless" in bed because fundamentally they feel guilty about being male.

97 *There's been a major shake-up in our sexual culture . . .* This may be true in certain parts of the developed West, but worldwide the bar for women's sexual satisfaction is still set very low. Hall and Graham's (2013) edited volume, *The Cultural Context of Sexual Pleasure and Problems*, vividly describes how traditional limitations on women's (and men's) sexual pleasure still persist in many, if not most, countries around the world.

99 *"I don't feel like a man anymore."* To quote Patricia Love and Steven Stosny, " 'Womanhood' is rarely at stake in sexual encounters, whereas 'manhood,' in the mind of the man at least, is very often at risk" (2007, p. 77).

Chapter 9: The Mysteries of Intercourse

103 *"Lord of Peace . . ."* This quotation from Rabbi Nachman (1772–1810) is today a bit of an anachronism. Women and men aren't really "opposites," and it's no longer considered accurate to refer to them as such.

105 *He is the hungry baby, and she is the all-giving mother.* See Dinnerstein (1976, p. 42).

108 *intercourse-related pain* Stein (2009) and Coady and Fish (2011) are both excellent guides to getting help for genital pain.

109 *trauma* A good book on sexual trauma such as Staci Haines's *Healing Sex* (2007) or Wendy Maltz's *The Sexual Healing Journey* (2012), or a therapist who's specifically trained in trauma work, can be invaluable.

Haines (2007, Chapter 3) is a useful guide to why dissociation happens, and what to do about it. Fonda (2014, pp. 28, 129) discusses "disembodiment/dissociation" in teenage girls who report that sex "just happened." (See also Tolman 2002, pp. 1–2.) Northrup (2010, p. 262) notes that many women accept intercourse when they only really want to be loved and receive sexual pleasure.

110 *Some men need very little stimulation to get off.* Often a partner will say, "Well, he got *his* pleasure." Not so. Sex is a bit like a meal, as we discussed in Chapter 6. A man with premature ejaculation sits down to eat, has a few bites of salad, then they clear everything away and bring him dessert and the check. Not very satisfying.

111 *stop-start* My go-to patient education resource on premature ejaculation is Michael Metz and Barry McCarthy's *Coping with Premature Ejaculation* (Metz and McCarthy, 2003). The authors are appropriately humble about the prognosis for remission of PE with stop/start, and they acknowledge the

merits of combining medication and behavioral treatments in men with severe symptoms. Helen Kaplan (1989) was more enthusiastic about stop-start-based methods—something I can only attribute to her never having had to struggle to hold back an orgasm.

PE can be a secondary symptom in men with a variety of conditions—from stress and anxiety to erectile dysfunction (Metz and McCarthy, 2003). But most men with rapid ejaculation have so-called primary PE, which is often lifelong. Such men often appear to be naturally endowed with very low ejaculation thresholds.

112 *"We are the most intensely excited . . ."* Morin (1995, p. 51).

113 *Sex-knots are the main reason sexual problems can be so difficult to fix.* Many authors have described similar patterns where each partner's natural reactions only make the situation worse (e.g., Love and Stosny 2007; Johnson 2008, 2013; Gottman and Silver 2015). My term for this, "sex-knots," was inspired by British psychiatrist R. D. Laing's book *Knots* (1972)—a gloomy little meditation on self-defeating cycles in human interactions. Unlike Laing's knots, the sex-knots you'll read about in this book can all be readily untied, once you know how.

116 *"outercourse"* Marty Klein and Riki Robbins's *Let Me Count the Ways* (1998) describes outercourse as *"both a set of erotic behaviors and an attitude towards them"* (p. 111). This "attitude" has some similarities to mindfulness practice (pp. 111–63).

Following Thomas Aquinas, for a long time it was taught that penis-vagina intercourse was the only kind of sexual activity that was in accordance with "natural law." This turns out not to be true.

Yes, penis-in-vagina sex is pretty standard in the animal kingdom. But there are lots of exceptions. According to Roughgarden (2013, p. 137) same-sex mating has been observed in over a hundred mammalian species. Male big-horned sheep (and many male domesticated sheep as well) prefer anal sex with other males (ibid., pp. 137–40). Male bottlenose dolphins will *shtup* any available orifice, and frequently form homosexual pairs (ibid., p. 141). Among our nearest relatives the bonobo apes, the most common sex act is probably genital rubbing between two females (ibid., pp. 148–50).

Among highly social primates like ourselves, most sexual encounters don't serve reproductive purposes as much as social ones—such as fostering harmony, strengthening emotional bonds, discharging aggression, and easing stress (ibid., pp. 149–50). Human sexuality becomes much easier to understand once you realize that its primary aims are social rather than strictly reproductive. For example, people debate why women have orgasms at all, since a woman's orgasm is not necessary for reproduction. But orgasms help cement social ties, and in a highly social species this has clear survival value—both for an individual and for her offspring.

118 *foreplay to "core-play"* Kerner (2004, Kindle ed. locations 528, 878, 894, and elsewhere). See also Lerner (2013, pp. 121–22).

Chapter 10: Why Women Lose Interest in Sex

119 *"I think about sex a lot . . ."* Hall (2004, p. 9). *Reclaiming Your Sexual Self* is my go-to patient education book for women struggling with low desire. It's one of the few sex books that takes the idea of a sexual self seriously.

120 *Most people . . . won't take their clothes off and mate with a near-stranger during their lunch hour for the sake of science . . .* As Leonore Tiefer discusses in *Sex Is Not a Natural Act* (2004), it took a particular kind of person to be willing to have sex with a stranger in a laboratory with instruments attached and cameras running (pp. 46–48).

120 *Helen Kaplan understood there was something missing from the Masters and Johnson model.* Kaplan (1995).

121 *The hydraulic model doesn't fit the facts of women's desire.* The most widely accepted theory of sexual desire these days is the *"incentive motivation model"* (Both, Everaerd, and Laan 2007), which holds that desire is primarily reactive to external stimuli rather than to anything internal. According to this model, what looks like spontaneous desire (e.g., frequent masturbation in a fourteen-year-old boy) is instead just extreme reactivity to environmental stimuli, including fantasy. See Toates (2014).

Arousal and desire may be fundamentally the same. In 2013, the American Psychiatric Association's DSM-5 Work Group for Sexual and Gender Identity Disorders concluded that there was insufficient evidence to distinguish disorders of female arousal from disorders of desire. Accordingly, a new unitary category was created: *Female Sexual Interest and Arousal Disorder (FSIAD)* (American Psychiatric Association 2013, p. 437).

121 *There are also lots of reasons a woman might not want to have sex.* My list is not intended to be comprehensive. More systematic listings may be found in Kaschak and Tiefer's *A New View of Women's Sexual Problems* (2001), or in Hall's *Reclaiming Your Sexual Self* (2004, pp. 38–64).

122 *Some women who've lost desire will keep having sex with their partner out of a sense of responsibility . . .* See Hall (2004, pp. 82–96) for an extensive discussion of the hazards of obligation sex, and some excellent alternative strategies.

Afterword
131 *Not all women who are as depressed as Marnie will get better just from couples therapy alone.* If a woman with depression and no desire for sex doesn't respond to individual or couple's therapy, then it's sometimes worth considering a careful trial of an

antidepressant. I often recommend bupropion, which is one of the few antidepressants without negative effects on libido.

In 2015 the FDA approved a nonhormonal agent, flibanserin (Addyi), for premenopausal women with "hypoactive sexual desire disorder." As of this writing few women have yet tried flibanserin, and it remains to be seen what role—if any—this new agent might have in the treatment of women like Marnie.

Chapter 11: Why Men Go Missing in Bed

133 *Most straight men tend to hear any female unhappiness as criticism.* According to Love and Stosny (2007), women and men tend to differ in what they dread most in relationships. Women tend to dread disconnection. This makes them want to reach out to their partners when they're in distress. Men tend to dread feeling inadequate, and hence often interpret their female partners' distress as an accusation that they've failed (pp. 1–27).

133 *"Many men are actually highly sensitive to evidence that their partners are unhappy . . ."* Bader (2009, p. 33).

134 *It's commonly assumed that men automatically want sex.* Most men also tend to use sex for emotional self-regulation. This adds to the impression that men are naturally horny all the time.

135 *Men get used to being the object of women's approval or disapproval when they are boys.* Girls obviously experience maternal disapproval as well, but they're more likely to *internalize* the disapproving voice. Men, on the other hand, often *externalize* it and try to get as far away from it as they can.

136 *Eventually . . . a man who feels criticized or unaccepted will usually just withdraw.* When a man withdraws from his partner sexually, he'll often turn to masturbation instead. Or rather, he'll *return* to it—since masturbation is where most men learn about sexual feelings in the first place.

Sexually, though, we're all like Pavlov's dog. If a man waits to go online until his wife falls asleep or leaves the house, over time, his sexual system will start to recognize her *absence* as a cue for sexual excitement. When her car pulls back into the driveway, that's now a cue to *shut down* arousal, delete the search history, and turn off desire. It's easy to see how this wouldn't be so great for married life.

139 *ADHD* Not all people with symptoms like David's turn out to have ADHD. There are many other conditions that can cause similar symptoms. It usually takes me about an hour or so of careful questioning to make the diagnosis with any degree of confidence.

My favorite kids' book on ADHD, *Jumpin' Johnny—Get Back to Work!* (Gordon 1998), begins with six words: "I just got yelled at again." That's it in a nutshell for many kids with this condition—and later for the adults they grow up to be.

Two very useful books on ADHD in adult relationships are *Is It You, Me, or Adult A.D.D.?* by Gina Pera (2008), and *The ADHD Effect on Marriage* by Melissa Orlov (2010). Both Pera and Orlov highlight the fact (Pera 2008, p. 56; Orlov 2010, p. 35) that some individuals with ADHD will tend to hyperfocus on a partner at the beginning of a relationship. This can lead to a severe let-down for the partner once courtship ends. Sometimes that's when the yelling starts.

ADHD also occurs in women, and the role adult ADHD plays in a woman's life can be both similar and different. People tend to assume that women will be more attentive, less distractible, and more adept at social interactions, so women often experience more shame about their symptoms (Kelly and Ramundo 2006, pp. 233–34; Solden 2005, pp. 55–118). Women also tend to be better at hiding their vulnerabilities, and are less likely to have a partner to organize their life (Solden 2005, p. 56).

By the way, there's now a mindfulness guide for people with ADHD (Zylowska, 2012).

141 *These days we therapists often refer to all these kinds of men as "atypical."* The informal term "atypical" derives from a term used in the Asperger's online community to describe non-Asperger individuals: "neuro-typical." Hence non-neuro-typical = atypical. Atypical might cover a gamut of developmental issues including ADHD, Specific Learning Disorders, Asperger's syndrome (or as it's known officially in psychiatry since 2013, "Autism Spectrum Disorder, Level 1"), Social (Pragmatic) Communication Disorder, Developmental Coordination Disorder, or problems with sensory integration and processing (Kranowitz 1998)—either alone, or more frequently in combination (Snyder, 2010; Kutscher, 2014). There are surely also other conditions as yet unnamed, and the universe of atypical individuals is no doubt broader than our current diagnostic categories might suggest.

There are books on living with an adult partner who has ADHD (Pera 2008; Orlov 2010) or autism spectrum (Aston 2011, 2013), and some memorable first-person accounts (e.g., Finch 2012). But I know of no relationship guides relevant to the broader universe of atypical adults with the other issues mentioned above. The pediatric self-help literature can be useful here (Kranowitz 1998; Kutscher 2014).

Avodah Offit, in a footnote to the revised 1983 edition of *The Sexual Self*, refers to a condition she calls "*'sexual dyskinesia' . . . lovers who are ineducably clumsy*" (p. 123). Marty Klein (2012, pp. 117–21) refers to this as a "neuro-sexual learning disability." The classic example is a man who despite having been given detailed instructions by his wife about how she'd like her clitoris stroked, can't seem to remember how to do it. The phenomenon is one of the most baffling in all of sexology. Is this really some kind of learning disability, or is he being passive-aggressive? Often both seem to be involved.

Klein (2012) notes that sometimes such an individual will have a partner who's *highly sensitive* to subtleties of touch (Kranowitz 1998). It can be important for a couple like this to understand that their primary difficulties are more neurological than emotional.

Chapter 12: Standing Your Ground

145 *"Sometimes . . . a man requires help . . ."* Offit (1981, p. 123).

Standing Your Ground

147 *David isn't backing down or apologizing.* Brown (2010, pp. 49–54) notes that in order to "stand on your sacred ground" you have to have sufficiently mastered your shame triggers. This was certainly the case with David.

149 *After years of watching families up close, Bowen felt he finally understood how families worked.* Kerr and Bowen (1988, pp. 6–14).

One weakness of Bowen Theory is that it doesn't account for neuropsychiatric influences on family interactions, but relies instead on social factors such as birth order to explain family patterns. In reality, a child's innate temperament and neuropsychiatric vulnerabilities tend to elicit specific and predictable responses from the rest of the family (Snyder 2010). See "Chipmunk Love," Chapter 11.

151 *Constructing the Sexual Crucible* Schnarch's 1991 book is still an excellent introduction to his thinking—and how it differs from the conventional Masters and Johnson model. But at 600-plus pages, it's suitable for only the most ardent professional reader.

Since then, Schnarch has written three books for lay audiences. *Passionate Marriage* (1997) is the best known. In his most recent book, *Intimacy and Desire* (2009), Schnarch describes four separate but interrelated aspects of differentiation that he calls "Four Points of Balance™" (Schnarch, 2009, pp. 72–74 and 85–89).

151 *"Marriage asks, 'Are you willing to stand up now . . . ?'"* Schnarch (2009, p. 232).

PART III: SEX FOR LIFE

Chapter 13: Eros and Faith

161 *You could define faith a million ways.* My approach to faith in Part III is principally derived from my own teacher Harold Bronheim's work on faith from an object relations psychoanalytic viewpoint (Bronheim 1998, pp. 18–44).

Faith often seems to be the product of having been sufficiently loved. So a secure and loving home life would seem to be crucial. But there are people of strong faith who had disastrous childhoods. And there are individuals from ordinarily loving families who because of some innate sensitivity in their wiring have nonetheless endured lasting damage to their faith.

The flip side of faith is connection to others, which as Bronheim (1998), Bader (2002), and Brown (2007, 2010) note puts faith in opposition to shame.

161 *"For myself I remember the kindness of your youth . . ."* The Bible is clear about the connection between divine love and erotic love. Whether it's the passage from Jeremiah quoted here, the entire *Song of Songs*, or numerous other places where prophets plead with the people not to run off to serve other gods, there is an explicit idea that the relationship between God and His people is like a sexually exclusive marriage. Or if you turn the equation the other way, that sex is an intimation of divine love.

164 *"introjects"* Introjects and other forms of internalization have traditionally been referred to as aspects of "internal object relations"—a term derived from early Freudian theory, which focused on how young children used the people around them as "objects" to satisfy physical needs. It's now recognized that even very young children's relationships to their caregivers are motivated by needs for attachment as well as physical gratification (Karen 1998; Lewis, Amini, and Lannon 2000; Johnson 2008, 2013).

169 *"The only thing that seems to help is when I tell you things that scare me."* For specific guidance on how to build your confidence as a couple by talking about difficult subjects, see Nelson (2008), Johnson (2008, 2013), and Gottman and Silver (2015).

Chapter 14: Becoming a Couple

173 *"The sexual is the most intimate world between two people . . ."* Offit (1983, p. 204).

173 *It's good to idealize your partner when you first fall in love.* Like sexual arousal, idealization of a partner in the first phase of love activates infantile feelings of having "everything." With any luck, further development of a love relationship eventually makes you feel you have "enough."

174 *inspiration, disappointment, and eventual creative mastery* I'm indebted to Akiva Tatz in *Living Inspired* (1993, pp. 17–28) for the insight that these are necessary stages in almost all human endeavors.

177 *. . . when a couple argues, they often have no idea what they're fighting about.* Lerner (2014, p. 37–38).

177 *Sometimes you have no idea who you're fighting with.* Lerner (2014, p. 154–88).

179 *triangles* For more on triangles, see Bowen (1978), Kerr and Bowen (1988), Gilbert (2013), and Lerner (2014). From the perspective of Bowen Theory, when you leave your parents and cleave unto your spouse, you're really only exchanging one set of triangles for another. There's so much ambivalence in human relationships that triangles seem to be necessary to keep them going. Religious people often have the advantage that a perceived relationship with God can be one corner of a triangle stabilizing a couple.

181 *"You're missing one of the great things about being gay . . ."* Sex advice columnist and author Dan Savage writes, *"Psychologists and psychiatrists used to argue that being gay was a choice your mother made for you. Mothers who were too close to their sons, mothers who 'smothered' their sons, risked turning them gay. The shrinks got it backward, mistaking one of the consequences of being gay—one of the perks of being gay—for the cause. The kind of relationship I had with my mother didn't make me gay. I had that kind of relationship with my mother because I was gay"* (2014, pp. 8–9).

Similarly, child psychoanalyst Ken Corbett notes that mothers play a particular and crucial role in fostering emotional resilience in their feminine sons (2009, pp. 114–15).

Chapter 15: Can Sex Survive Monogamy?

185 *"My experience indicates that most people become infatuated . . ."* Offit (1983, p. 227).

188 *Your sexual self doesn't understand the whole monogamy thing at all.* Offit (1981, pp. 45–46) notes that there are at least fourteen predictable moments in a marriage when sexual infidelity is most likely to occur. These include several that are relevant here: being heavily involved in expansion or success, traveling extensively alone, times of bereavement, and times when one confronts the realities of physically aging.

188 *Strict sexual monogamy is a fairly recent development in human history.* For most of human history our ancestors were nomads who probably shared everything—including sex partners. As discussed in Notes to Chapter 4, strict sexual monogamy may have been a by-product of the agricultural revolution (Ryan and Jetha 2010).

188 *Not everyone opts for monogamy.* Many sex writers have wondered whether strict sexual monogamy might now no longer be necessary—especially because so many people fail at it anyway—and whether some couples might do better with mutually negotiated open relationships (Brandon 2010; Nelson 2012). There's been some extremely interesting work on the ethics of this—from occasional "dalliances" (Morin, 1995; see also Savage 2014) to full-on polyamory (Easton and Hardy, 2009; Veaux and Rickert, 2014; Jenkins, 2017).

Most writers on the subject agree that it takes time and energy to deal with the complex feelings that can arise in open relationships. This can be a serious issue in our day, when most couples hardly have time and energy for even *one* sexual relationship.

Most discussions of non-monogamy don't take into full account the feelings of the third person involved. This is an important omission. Veaux and Rickert in *More Than Two* point out that most open relationships are structured to protect the primary couple at the expense of the third, who can end up being treated as a "need-fulfillment machine" rather than as a full person (2014, pp. 180–218).

Most couples I know who have happy, mutually negotiated open relationships are either gay men in "monogamish" unions (Savage 2014), people who are into kink (once you've crossed one sexual boundary, the others somehow tend not to look so imposing), or older couples who have the time, energy, and maturity for such things and whose kids have left the house. (There's little doubt in my mind that the next sexual revolution will be led by retirees.)

Most other people seem to value strict sexual monogamy, or at least say they do, or are bound to do so for religious reasons. My main intent in Part III is to provide such couples with strategies for how to succeed in sexually exclusive relationships. For other couples, Easton Hardy (2009) and Veaux and Rickert (2014) might serve as a good introduction to the possibilities and challenges of open relationships—though as Veaux and Rickert point out (ibid., p. 2), it's too early to call anyone an expert on this yet.

189 *The erotic mind doesn't handle loss very well.* I'm indebted here to Daniel Watter and Esther Perel, both of whom independently gave presentations at a recent SSTAR meeting on the role of grief and loss in infidelity (Perel, 2013; Watter, 2013).

194 *Emily wonders whether it might help to get her body moving.* Given the many women who seem to need to reconnect with their bodies in order to feel sexual, many people have wondered whether some women might have an innate vulnerability to disconnection, which is then reinforced in an antisexual culture. In the laboratory, women tend to have lower *concordance* between subjective sexual excitement and objective measures of genital arousal, and there is evidence that women with sexual dysfunctions show even lower concordance than women without sexual dysfunction (Chivers et al. 2010). Brotto et al. (2016b) found that Mindfulness-Based Sex Therapy (MBST) improved concordance in women presenting with sexual desire/arousal difficulties.

Chapter 16: Mindfulness, Heartfulness, and Prayer

199 *More Than Two* The title of this section is taken from Veaux and Rickert (2014).

202 *"When my beloved first stands before me naked . . ."* Peck (1978, p. 181).

Most readers of *The Road Less Traveled* probably never guessed that Peck's "beloved" in the quote above might not have been his wife. Earlier in the book, tucked away in a footnote, Peck had written the following: *"My work with couples has led me to the stark conclusion that open marriage is the only kind of mature marriage that is healthy and not seriously destructive to the spiritual health and growth of the individual partners"* (Peck, 1978, p. 93). The "open marriage" movement of the 1970s quietly wound down when it encountered AIDS and the Reagan era. But there are signs of its revival today, as discussed in Notes to Chapter 15.

203 *I think every erotic couple eventually develops a private religion of their own* . . . "Creating shared meaning" is the last of Gottman and Silver's *Seven Principles for Making Marriage Work* (2015, pp. 260–76).

203 *A more sensible definition of prayer* . . . I'm indebted to Akiva Tatz (1993, p. 104) for this insight.

203 *Great sex, like deep prayer, can be an act of surrender.* Gina Ogden's *The Heart and Soul of Sex* (2006) and *The Return of Desire* (2008) contain a variety of first-person accounts from people who report having had transcendent or life-changing experiences while making love. Kleinplatz et al. (2009) contains several others.

204 *"peak erotic experiences"* Morin (1995).

Sex writers vary in their attitudes toward "great sex" in long-term relationships. Schnarch (1991, 1997) unabashedly celebrates it, but states that few people are willing to risk the raw intimacy it takes to get there. Morin (1995), borrowing from Maslow (1967, 1971), writes about using one's own past "peak erotic experiences" as a guide to self-understanding—but most of the peak experiences he discusses don't happen within ongoing committed relationships.

In 2006 a research group headed by Peggy Kleinplatz began interviewing dozens of people who self-identified as having great sex in long-term relationships, to find out what exactly they were describing and whether it might be useful to couples in general (Kleinplatz et al. 2009a, 2009b, 2013; Menard 2015). Kleinplatz's participants were a self-selected group. But their descriptions were remarkably consistent with each other. The ingredients for "great sex" identified by this group were primarily emotional rather than physical, and included such qualities as "authenticity," "vulnerability," and "being present."

Many of Kleinplatz's participants were in monogamous relationships of thirty years or more. Others were in consensually non-monogamous relationships and/or self-identified as LGBT or kinky. Kleinplatz has argued that couples in general can learn much from members of sexual minorities about how to have deeper, more meaningful erotic experiences (Kleinplatz 2006).

Other writers (e.g., Zilbergeld, 1992; Metz and McCarthy 2012; Klein 2012) deemphasize the pursuit of "great sex" and tend to focus instead on helping couples just relax and enjoy ordinarily good sex. David Scharff, echoing British pediatrician and psychoanalyst D. W. Winnicott's notion of the "good enough mother" (Winnicott 1965), discussed the idea of "good enough sex" (Scharff, 1982, p. 10; see also Scharff and Scharff 1991, p. 13). Later, Barry McCarthy and Michael Metz made "Good Enough Sex" the centerpiece of a philosophy of unpressured lovemaking (Metz and McCarthy, 2012).

I prefer "The Sanctification of the Ordinary." Not only does it sound more inspiring, but I also think "sanctification" is the most accurate term to describe what most happily committed couples do when they make love.

Getting Practical: Sex Tune-Ups for Couples

204 *"sensate focus"* Weiner and Avery-Clark's *Sensate Focus in Sex Therapy: The Illustrated Manual* (2017) is an invaluable resource for therapists wishing to learn this technique.

Technically speaking, the practices described in Chapter 16 all fall under what Weiner and Avery-Clark, following Masters and Johnson, refer to as "Sensate Focus 1." Couples then move on to "Sensate Focus 2," where they're encouraged to provide each other with verbal and nonverbal information about their feelings, preferences, wants, and needs.

The practice that I refer to as "taking touch" is referred to by Weiner and Avery-Clark as "non-demand touching for one's own interest" or "non-demand touching for self." I prefer "taking touch" since it emphasizes the selfish aspect, which for many couples is somewhat foreign.

Sensate Focus 1 is designed to be very different from an ordinary romantic or erotic encounter. All touching is done with the hands only; at first there's no kissing or full-body contact; and couples are encouraged to focus specifically on the *"temperature* (cool or warm), *pressure* (hard or soft), and *texture* (smooth or rough)" of the part being touched (Weiner and Avery-Clark, 2014)—aspects of the experience that are intended to be "neutral" and low in emotional intensity.

Many couples complain that sensate focus feels too "clinical" or "sterile"—which often indicates that no one ever fully explained its rationale to them. As Weiner and Avery-Clark (2014) note, sensate focus is less a practice than an *attitude.* This attitude can feel odd and unfamiliar at first, but it can be learned.

205 *Pleasure is an emotion, and you can't control emotions.* Weiner and Avery-Clark (2014).

206 *Part of the field's renewed interest in sensate focus may have to do with the fact that it's essentially a mindfulness practice.* See Brotto and Goldmeier (2015).

Chapter 17 Care of the Sexual Soul

207 *"If love is a place, even if it's a scary place, I want to live there."* Doyle (2016, p. 191).

211 *"I thought that was just the way it was."* Bader (2002) writes movingly about how children adapt to adverse early environments: *"If we can avoid or repair a rupture in our relationships with our parents by suppressing or altering our feelings, desires, and even our perceptions, we will do it instinctively, naturally, without a conscious thought"* (p. 20).

Seen from this perspective, the ability to selfishly "use" someone you love for your own pleasure can be a tremendous achievement. Again quoting Bader, *"I am not talking about actually disregarding the feelings of the other but about a quality of relatedness in which the other does not need to be taken care of and, thus, can be taken for granted.... One patient described the most intense moments of her sexual excitement as feeling like waves crashing up against a shore that is steady, sturdy, and unyielding. She didn't have to worry about whether the 'shore' could take it"* (p. 33). In *The Deep Yes* (2016), Rosalyn Dischiavo writes about being able to relax into an attitude of deep, unworried *receiving*—which I believe is ultimately the same thing.

215 *Sarina drifts along in her river of sadness.* Technically speaking, Sarina didn't follow standard technique for Sensate Focus 1 when she allowed herself to be swept away by emotion instead of redirecting her focus to the pressure, temperature, and texture of Jo's touch (Weiner and Avery-Clark 2014, 2017—see Notes to Chapter 16). And Jo didn't follow the standard prescription to limit herself to using only her hands. Rather than adhere to the

standard procedure, I chose to follow Sarina and Jo's intuitive preference for a more emotionally charged experience.

Chapter 18: Childhood's End

217 *Tantra* Ritual sex was only one of the ways that Tantric practice was a radical departure from ordinary high-caste Hindu behavior. The others included eating meat and fish, and drinking wine and fermented grain (Brooks 1990, pp. 69–70; Sanderson 1988, pp. 661–62). But here in the West, the word "Tantra" has now become more or less synonymous with ritual sex.

220 *"To go to a funeral is to have sex afterward, if you can . . ."* Offit (1983, p. 23).

223 *"The touch of mother's arms, breasts, and body had to be an early ecstasy for which we search again . . ."* Offit (1983, p. 21).

223 *"Some people just seem to have a knack for being alone."* Psychological research on mother-child attachment is now over fifty years old and from the start has been an extraordinarily complex project. See Robert Karen's *Becoming Attached* (1998) for more information about the experiment described here, and for an account of subsequent developments in this line of research (pp. 143–61 and subsequent chapters).

As Karen notes, people with attachment-related issues vary *"from people who are essentially whole but have certain types of struggles in the realm of intimacy to those who are so badly damaged by crazy, violent, depressed, rejecting or absent parents that they were never able to internalize enough sense of goodness about them-selves and others to keep rage, paranoia, and panic from spoiling their lives"* (p. 390). My "Emily" clearly represents the former type: someone "essentially whole," but with attachment-related intimacy issues.

For more on adult attachment issues, see Lewis, Amini, and

Lannon (2000); Johnson (2008, 2013); Levine and Heller (2010); and Resnick (2012).

225 *"The windows across the courtyard are glowing . . ."* Offit (1981, pp. 14–15).

Appendix: Eleven Sex-Knots, and How to Untie Them

229 *As the Buddhist sage Shunryu Suzuki taught . . .* Many versions of this saying of Suzuki's have found their way into circulation. The canonical version seems to be, *"In zazen (sitting meditation), leave your front door and back door open. Let thoughts come and go. Just don't serve them tea."* (Chadwick, 1999, p. 301).

Sources

American Association of Sex Educators, Counselors, and Therapists. AASECT Code of Ethics. Washington, DC: AASECT, 1978.

American Psychiatric Association. *Diagnostic and Statistical Manual for Mental Disorders, Fifth Edition.* Arlington, VA: American Psychiatric Association, 2013.

Aston, Maxine. *The Other Half of Asperger Syndrome: A Guide to Living in an Intimate Relationship with a Partner Who Has Asperger Syndrome.* London: National Autistic Society, 2001.

———. *Aspergers in Love: Couple Relationships and Family Affairs.* London: Jessica Kingsley, 2003.

Bader, Michael J. *Arousal: The Secret Logic of Sexual Fantasies.* New York: Thomas Dunne, 2002.

———. *Male Sexuality: Why Women Don't Understand It—and Men Don't Either.* Lanham, MD: Rowman & Littlefield, 2009.

Bancroft, John. *Human Sexuality and Its Problems*, 3rd ed. Edinburgh, UK: Churchill Livingstone/Elsevier, 2009.

Bancroft, John, Cynthia A. Graham, Erick Janssen, and Stephanie A. Sanders.

"The Dual Control Model: Current Status and Future Directions." *Journal of Sex Research* 46 (2009): 121–42.

Barbach, Lonnie. *For Yourself: The Fulfillment of Female Sexuality.* Garden City, NY: Doubleday, 1975.

Barmak, Sarah. *Closer: Notes from the Orgasmic Frontier of Female Sexuality.* Toronto: Coach House Books, 2016.

Benjamin, Jessica. *The Bonds of Love: Psychoanalysis, Feminism, and the Problem of Domination.* New York: Pantheon, 1988.

Bogaert, Anthony F., and Lori Brotto, "Object of Desire Self-Consciousness Theory." *Journal of Sex and Marital Therapy* 40, no. 4 (2014): 323–38.

Bogaert, Anthony F., Beth A. Visser, Julie A. Pozzebon. "Gender Differences in Object of Desire Self-Consciousness Sexual Fantasies." *Archives of Sexual Behavior* 44, no. 8 (2015): 2299–310.

Both, Stephanie, Walter Everaerd, and Ellen Laan. "Desire Emerges from Excitement: A Psychophysiological Perspective on Sexual Motivation." In *The Psychophysiology of Sex*, edited by Erick Janssen. Bloomington: Indiana University Press, 2007.

Bowen, Murray. *Family Therapy in Clinical Practice.* New York: Jason Aronson, 1978.

Brandon, Marianne. *Monogamy: The Untold Story.* Santa Barbara, CA: Praeger, 2010.

Bronheim, Harold E. *Body and Soul: The Role of Object Relations in Faith, Shame, and Healing.* Northvale, NJ: Jason Aronson, 1998.

Brooks, Douglas Renfrew. *The Secret of the Three Cities: An Introduction to Hindu Śākta Tantrism.* Chicago: University of Chicago Press, 1990.

Brotto, Lori. "Mindfulness Based Cognitive Therapy for Women with Low Desire, Sexual Pain or Histories of Sexual Trauma." Center for Love and Sex (Sari Cooper, Director). New York, NY. November 4, 2016a.

Brotto, Lori A., and Rosemary Basson. "Group Mindfulness-Based Therapy Significantly Improves Sexual Desire in Women." *Behavioural Research and Therapy* 57 (2014): 143–54.

Brotto, Lori A., Meredith L. Chivers, Roanne D. Millman, and Arianne Albert. "Mindfulness-Based Sex Therapy Improves Genital-Subjective Arousal Concordance in Women with Sexual Desire/Arousal Difficulties." *Archives of Sexual Behavior* 45, no. 8 (2016b): 1907–21.

Brotto, Lori, and David Goldmeier. "Mindfulness Interventions for

Treating Sexual Dysfunctions: The Gentle Science of Finding Focus in a Multitask World." *Journal of Sexual Medicine* 12 no. 8 (2015): 1687–89.

Brown, Brené. *I Thought It Was Just Me (But It Isn't)*. New York: Avery, 2007.

———. *The Gifts of Imperfection*. Center City, MN: Hazelden, 2010.

Carpenter, Deanna, Erick Janssen, Cynthia Graham, Harrie Vorst, and Jelte Wicherts. "Women's Scores on the Sexual Inhibition/Sexual Excitation Scales (SIS/SES): Gender Similarities and Differences." *Journal of Sex Research* 45, no. 1 (2008): 36–48.

Chadwick, David. *Crooked Cucumber: The Life and Zen Teaching of Shunryu Suzuki*. New York: Broadway Books, 1999.

Chalker, Rebecca. *The Clitoral Truth*. New York: Seven Stories Press, 2000.

Chivers, Meredith L., Michael C. Seto, Martin L. Lalumiere, Ellen Laan, Teresa Grimbos. "Agreement of Self-Reported and Genital Measures of Sexual Arousal in Men and Women: A Meta-Analysis." *Archives of Sexual Behavior* 39 (2010): 5–56.

Coady, Deborah, and Nancy Fish. *Healing Painful Sex: A Woman's Guide to Confronting, Diagnosing, and Treating Sexual Pain*. Berkeley, CA: Seal, 2011.

Cohn, Ruth. *Coming Home to Passion—Restoring Loving Sexuality in Couples with Histories of Childhood Trauma and Neglect*. Santa Barbara, CA: Praeger, 2011.

Corbett, Ken. *Boyhoods: Rethinking Masculinities*. New Haven, CT: Yale University Press, 2009.

Daedone, Nicole. *Slow Sex: The Art and Craft of the Female Orgasm*. New York: Grand Central, 2011.

Dederer, Claire. "Why Is It So Hard for Women to Write About Sex?" *The Atlantic*. March 2014.

———. *Love and Trouble: A Midlife Reckoning*. New York: Alfred A. Knopf, 2017.

Dinnerstein, Dorothy. *The Mermaid and the Minotaur: Sexual Arrangements and Human Malaise*. New York: Other, 1999. First published 1976 by Harper and Row.

Dischiavo, Rosalyn. *The Deep Yes: The Lost Art of True Receiving*. Spanda Press, 2016.

Doyle, Glennon. *Love Warrior*. New York: Flatiron Books, 2016.

Drescher, Jack. "Out of DSM: Depathologizing Homosexuality." *Behavioral Sciences* 5 (2015): 565–75.

Drescher, Jack, and Joseph P. Merlino, eds. *American Psychiatry and Homosexuality: An Oral History*. New York: Routledge 2007.

Easton, Dossie, and Janet W. Hardy. *The Ethical Slut: A Practical Guide to Polyamory, Open Relationships & Other Adventures*, 2nd ed. Berkeley, CA: Celestial Arts, 2009.

Federation of Feminist Women's Health Centers. *A New View of a Woman's Body*. New York: Touchstone, 1981.

Feeney, Katherine. "Saying Yes to the Female Orgasm." *Sydney Morning Herald*, April 24, 2014.

Fertel, Evan. "Who Is This About? An Exploratory Study of Erotic Self-Focus" (2015). *UNLV Theses, Dissertations, Professional Papers, and Capstones*. Available for download at: http://digitalscholarship.unlv.edu/thesesdissertations/2349.

Finch, David. *The Journal of Best Practices: A Memoir of Marriage, Asperger Syndrome, and One Man's Quest to Be a Better Husband*. New York: Scribner, 2012.

Foley, Sallie, Sally A. Kope, and Dennis P. Sugrue. *Sex Matters for Women: A Complete Guide to Taking Care of Your Sexual Self*, 2nd ed. New York: Guilford Press, 2011.

Fonda, Jane. *Being a Teen: Everything Teen Girls and Boys Should Know about Relationships, Sex, Love, Health, Identity & More*. New York: Random House, 2014.

Freud, Sigmund. *Three Essays on the Theory of Sexuality* (1905). In *The Standard Edition of the Complete Psychological Works of Sigmund Freud*. Vol. VII, edited by James Strachey. London: Hogarth Press, 1966.

———. *On Narcissism: An Introduction* (1914). In *The Standard Edition of the Complete Psychological Works of Sigmund Freud*. Vol. XIV, edited by James Strachey. London: Hogarth Press, 1966.

Friday, Nancy. *My Secret Garden: Women's Sexual Fantasies*. New York: Pocket Books, 1973.

Gallwey, W. Timothy. *The Inner Game of Tennis*. New York: Random House, 1974.

Gartner, Richard B. *Betrayed as Boys: Psychodynamic Treatment of Sexually Abused Men*. New York: Guilford, 1999.

———. *Beyond Betrayal: Taking Charge of Your Life after Boyhood Sexual Abuse*. Hoboken, NJ: John Wiley & Sons, 2005.

Gilbert, Roberta M. *The Eight Concepts of Bowen Theory*. Falls Church, VA: Leading Systems Press, 2013.

Gordon, Michael. *Jumpin' Johnny Get Back to Work! A Child's Guide to ADHD/Hyperactivity*. DeWitt, NY: GSI Publications, 1998.

Gottlieb, Lori. "Does a More Equal Marriage Mean Less Sex?" *New York Times Magazine*, February 6, 2014.

Gottman, John M., and Nan Silver. *The Seven Principles for Making Marriage Work*, 2nd ed. New York: Harmony Books, 2015. First published 1999.

Graham, Cynthia A., Stephanie A. Sanders, and Robin R. Millhausen. "The Sexual Excitation/Sexual Inhibition Inventory for Women: Psychometric Properties." *Archives of Sexual Behavior* 35, no. 4 (2006): 397–409.

Gray, John. *Men Are from Mars, Women Are from Venus*. 20th Anniversary paperback ed. New York: HarperCollins, 2012. First published 1992.

Haines, Staci. *Healing Sex: A Mind-Body Approach to Healing Sexual Trauma*, 2nd ed. San Francisco: Cleis Press, 2007.

Hall, Kathryn. *Reclaiming Your Sexual Self: How You Can Bring Desire Back into Your Life*. Hoboken, NJ: John Wiley & Sons, 2004.

Hall, Kathryn S. K., and Cynthia A. Graham, eds. *The Cultural Context of Sexual Pleasure and Problems: Psychotherapy with Diverse Clients*. New York: Routledge, 2013.

Heiman, Julia, and Joseph LoPiccolo. *Becoming Orgasmic: A Sexual and Personal Growth Program for Women*. New York: Simon & Schuster, 1992. First published 1976 by Prentice-Hall.

Jannini, Emmanuele A., Odile Buisson, and Alberto Rubio-Casillas. Beyond the G-Spot: Clitourethrovaginal Complex Anatomy in Female Orgasm. *Nature Reviews Urology* 11 (2014): 531–38.

Janssen, Erick, and John Bancroft. "The Dual Control Model: The Role of Sexual Inhibition and Excitation in Sexual Arousal and Behavior." In *The Psychophysiology of Sex*. Bloomington: Indiana University Press, 2007.

Jenkins, Carrie. *What Love Is: And What It Could Be*. New York: Basic Books, 2017.

Joannides, Paul. *Guide to Getting It On! Unzipped.* Goofy Foot Press, 2017.

Johnson, Susan M. *Hold Me Tight: Seven Conversations for a Lifetime of Love.* New York: Little, Brown, 2008.

———. *Love Sense: The Revolutionary New Science of Romantic Relationships.* New York: Little, Brown, 2013.

Joyce, James. *Ulysses.* Paris: Shakespeare and Company, 1922.

Kabat-Zinn, Jon. *Mindfulness for Beginners.* Boulder, CO: Sounds True, 2012.

Kahn, Michael D. "Through a Glass Brightly: Treating Sexual Intimacy as the Restoration of the Whole Person." In *Intimate Environments: Sex, Intimacy, and Gender in Families,* edited by David Kantor and Barbara F. Okun. New York: Guilford Press, 1989.

Kaplan, Helen Singer. *The New Sex Therapy; Active Treatment of Sexual Dysfunctions.* New York: Times Books, 1974.

———. *PE: How to Overcome Premature Ejaculation.* New York: Routledge, 1994. First published 1989.

———. *The Sexual Desire Disorders.* New York: Routledge, 1995.

Karen, Robert. *Becoming Attached: First Relationships and How They Shape Our Capacity to Love.* New York: Oxford University Press, 1998.

Kaschak, Ellyn, and Leonore Tiefer, eds. *A New View of Women's Sexual Problems.* New York: Routledge, 2013. First published 2001 by Haworth Press.

Kelly, Kate, and Peggy Ramundo. *You Mean I'm Not Lazy, Stupid or Crazy?! A Classic Self-Help Book for Adults with Attention Deficit Disorder.* New York: Scribner, 2006.

Kerner, Ian. *She Comes First: The Thinking Man's Guide to Pleasuring a Woman.* New York: Regan, 2004.

Kerr, Michael E., and Murray Bowen. *Family Evaluation: An Approach Based on Bowen Theory.* New York: W.W. Norton, 1988.

Klein, Marty. *Sexual Intelligence: What We Really Want from Sex—and How to Get It.* New York: HarperOne, 2012.

Klein, Marty, and Riki Robbins. *Let Me Count the Ways—Discovering Great Sex Without Intercourse.* New York: Jeremy P. Tarcher/Putnam, 1998.

Kleinplatz, Peggy J. "Learning from Extraordinary Lovers: Lessons from the Edge." *Journal of Homosexuality* 50 (2006): 325–48.

Kleinplatz, Peggy J., A. Dana Menard, Marie-Pierre Paquet, Nicolas Paradis, Meghan Campbell, Dino Zuccarino, and Lisa Mehak. "The Components of Optimal Sexuality: A Portrait of 'Great Sex.'" *Canadian Journal of Human Sexuality* 18 (2009a): 1–13.

Kleinplatz, Peggy J. A. Dana Menard, Nicolas Paradis, Meghan Campbell, and Tracy Dalgleish. "Beyond Sexual Stereotypes: Revealing Group Similarities and Differences in Optimal Sexuality." *Canadian Journal of Behavioural Sciences* 45 (2013): 250–58.

Kleinplatz, Peggy J., A. Dana Menard, Nicolas Paradis, Meghan Campbell, Tracy Delgleish, Andrew Segovia, and Kellie Davis. "From Closet to Reality: Optimal Sexuality Among the Elderly." *The Irish Psychiatrist* 10 (2009b): 15–18.

Kocsis, Agnes, and John Newbury-Helps. "Mindfulness in Sex Therapy and Intimate Relationships (MSIR): Clinical Protocol and Theory Development." *Mindfulness* 7, no. 3 (2016): 690–99.

Kort, Joe, and Alexander P. Morgan. *Is My Husband Gay, Straight, or Bi? A Guide for Women Concerned About Their Men.* Lanham, MD: Rowman and Littlefield, 2014.

Kranowitz, Carol Stock. *The Out-of-Sync Child.* New York: Penguin, 2005. First published 1998 by Perigee.

Kutscher, Martin L. *Kids in the Syndrome Mix of ADHD, LD, Autism Spectrum, Tourette's, Anxiety, and More,* 2nd ed. London: Jessica Kingsley Publishers, 2014.

Laing, R. D. *Knots.* New York: Vintage Books, 1972.

Lamb, David. "Fictional Photographer Is Larger Than Life: National Geographic Has Been Busy Setting the Record Straight that 'Bridges' Character Robert Kincaid Doesn't Exist." *Los Angeles Times,* June 20, 1995. Accessed July 17, 2017 online: http://articles.latimes.com/1995-06-20/news/mn-15025_1_robert-kincaid.

Lamott, Anne. *Plan B: Further Thoughts on Faith.* New York: Riverhead Books, 2005.

Lerner, Harriet. *The Dance of Anger: A Woman's Guide to Changing the Patterns of Intimate Relationships.* New York: William Morrow, 2014. First published 1985 by Harper and Row.

———. *Marriage Rules: A Manual for the Married and the Coupled Up.* New York: Avery, 2013.

Lewis, Thomas, Fari Amini, and Richard Lannon. *A General Theory of Love*. New York: Vintage Books, 2000.

Love, Patricia, and Steven Stosny. *How to Improve Your Marriage Without Talking About It*. New York: Broadway Books, 2007.

Madsen, Pamela. *Shameless: How I Ditched the Diet, Got Naked, Found True Pleasure . . . and Somehow Got Home in Time to Cook Dinner*. New York: Rodale, 2011.

———. "How Women Are Enjoying Their Own Sexual Renaissance." *Huffington Post*, December 20, 2016.

Maier, Thomas. *Masters of Sex*. New York: Basic Books, 2009.

Maltz, Wendy. *The Sexual Healing Journey: A Guide for Survivors of Sexual Abuse*, 3rd ed. New York: HarperCollins, 2012.

Maslow, Abraham H. *Religions, Values, and Peak-Experiences*. New York: Viking, 1967.

———. *The Farther Reaches of Human Nature*. New York: Viking, 1971.

Meana, Marta. "Elucidating Women's (Hetero)Sexual Desire: Definitional Challenges and Content Expansion." *Journal of Sex Research* 47 (2010): 104–22.

Meana, Marta, and Evan Fertel. Plenary address: "It's Not You, It's Me. Exploring Erotic Self-Focus." 41st Annual Meeting, Society for Sex Therapy and Research. Chicago, Illinois, April 16, 2016.

Menard, A. Dana, Peggy J. Kleinplatz, Lianne Rosen, Shannon Lawless, Nicholas Paradis, Meghan Campbell, and Jonathan D. Huber. "Individual and Relational Contributors to Optimal Sexual Experiences in Older Men and Women." *Sexual and Relationship Therapy* 30, no. 1 (2015): 78–93.

Metz, Michael E., and Barry W. McCarthy. *Coping with Premature Ejaculation*. Oakland, CA: New Harbinger Publications, 2003.

———. "The Good Enough Sex (GES) model." In *New Directions in Sex Therapy*, 2nd ed., edited by Peggy Kleinplatz, 213–30. New York: Routledge, 2012.

Morin, Jack. *The Erotic Mind: Unlocking the Inner Sources of Sexual Passion and Fulfillment*. New York: HarperCollins, 1995.

Mosher, Donald L. "Three Dimensions of Depth of Involvement in Human Sexual Response." *Journal of Sex Research* 16 (1980): 1–42.

Nagoski, Emily. *Come as You Are: The Surprising New Science That Will Transform Your Sex Life*. New York: Simon & Schuster, 2015.

Nelson, Tammy. *Getting the Sex You Want*. Beverly, MA: Quiver, 2008.

————. *The New Monogamy: Redefining Your Relationship after Infidelity.* Oakland, CA: New Harbinger, 2012.

Nichols, Margaret. "Same-Sex Sexuality from a Global Perspective." In *The Cultural Context of Sexual Pleasure and Problems*, edited by Kathryn S.K. Hall and Cynthia A. Graham, 23–46. New York: Routledge, 2013.

————. "Therapy with LGBTQ Clients: Working with Sex and Gender Variance from a Queer Theory Model." In *Principles and Practice of Sex Therapy*, 5th ed., edited by Yitzchak M. Binik and Kathryn S.K. Hall, 309–33. New York: Guilford Press, 2014.

Northrup, Christiane. *Women's Bodies, Women's Wisdom*, rev. ed. New York: Bantam Books, 2010. First published 1994.

Offit, Avodah K. *The Sexual Self*. New York: Congdon & Weed, 1983. First published 1977 by J. B. Lippincott.

————. *Night Thoughts: Reflections of a Sex Therapist*. New York: Congdon & Lattes, 1981.

Ogas, Ogi, and Sai Gaddam. *A Billion Wicked Thoughts: What the World's Largest Experiment Reveals about Human Desire*. New York: Dutton, 2011.

Ogden, Gina. *The Heart and Soul of Sex*. Boston: Trumpeter, 2006.

————. *The Return of Desire*. Boston: Trumpeter, 2008.

Orenstein, Peggy. *Girls & Sex: Navigating the Complicated New Landscape*. New York: HarperCollins, 2016.

Orlov, Melissa. *The ADHD Effect on Marriage*. Plantation, FL: Specialty Press, 2010.

Peck, M. Scott. *The Road Less Traveled: A New Psychology of Love, Traditional Values, and Spiritual Growth*. New York: Simon and Schuster, 1978.

Pera, Gina. *Is It You, Me, or Adult A.D.D.?* San Francisco: 1201 Alarm Press, 2008.

Perel, Esther. *Mating in Captivity: Reconciling the Erotic and the Domestic*. New York: HarperCollins, 2006.

————. "The Double Flame: Reconciling Intimacy and Sexuality, Reviving Desire." In *Treating Sexual Desire Disorders: A Clinical Casebook*, edited by Sandra R. Leiblum, 23–43. New York: Guilford Press, 2010.

————. Paper presentation: "The State of Affairs—Rethinking Our Clinical Attitudes About Infidelity." SSTAR 38th Annual Meeting, Baltimore, April 6, 2013.

Pickert, Kate. "The Mindful Revolution." *Time* February 3, 2014.

Pogrebin, Letty C. "I Still Have Great Sex with My Husband and We've Been Married for 37 Years." *Elle* (online), March 27, 2016.

Réage, Pauline. *Story of O.* Paris: chez jean-jacques fauvert, 1954.

Resnick, Stella. *The Heart of Desire: Keys to the Pleasures of Love.* Hoboken, NJ: John Wiley & Sons, 2012.

Roughgarden, Joan. *Evolution's Rainbow: Diversity, Gender, and Sexuality in Nature and People,* 10th ed. Berkeley: University of California Press, 2013. First published 2004.

Ryan, Christopher, and Cacilda Jetha. *Sex at Dawn.* New York: Harper-Collins, 2010.

Sanderson, Alexis. "Śaivism and the Tantric Traditions." In *The World's Religions,* edited by Stewart Sutherland, Leslie Houlden, Peter Clarke, and Friedhelm Hardy. London: Routledge, 1988.

Savage, Dan. *American Savage.* New York: Plume, 2014.

Savin-Williams, Ritch C. "How Many Straight People Are There?" *Psychology Today* (online), July 4, 2016.

Scharff, David E. *The Sexual Relationship: An Object Relations View of Sex and the Family.* Boston: Routledge and Kegan Paul, 1982.

Scharff, David E., and Jill Savege Scharff. *Object Relations Couple Therapy.* Lanham, MD: Jason Aronson/Rowman and Littlefield, 1991.

Schiavo, Rosalyn. *The Deep Yes: The Lost Art of True Receiving.* Spanda Press, 2016.

Schnarch, David M. *Constructing the Sexual Crucible: An Integration of Sexual and Marital Therapy.* New York: W. W. Norton, 1991.

———. *Passionate Marriage.* New York: Henry Holt, 1998. First published 1997 by W. W. Norton.

———. *Intimacy & Desire.* New York: Beaufort Books, 2009.

Segal, Zindel, Mark Williams, and John Teasdale. *Mindfulness-Based Cognitive Therapy for Depression,* 2nd ed. New York: Guilford Press, 2013.

Serano, Julia. *Whipping Girl: A Transsexual Woman on Sexism and the Scapegoating of Femininity.* Berkeley, CA: Seal Press, 2007.

Snyder, Stephen. Clinical presentation: "All Kinds of Sexual Minds." SSTAR Fall Clinical Meeting, New York, 2010. (Avodah Offit, discussant).

———. Review of *Slow Sex: The Art and Craft of the Female Orgasm* by Nicole Daedone. *Journal of Sex & Marital Therapy* 39 (2012): 195–97.

Solden, Sari. *Women with Attention Deficit Disorder*. Ann Arbor, MI: Introspect Press, 2005.

Stein, Amy. *Heal Pelvic Pain*. New York: McGraw-Hill, 2009.

Tatz, Akiva. *Living Inspired*. Southfield, MI: Targum, 1993.

Tiefer, Leonore. *Sex Is Not a Natural Act, and Other Essays*. Boulder, CO: Westview, 2004.

———. "Sex Therapy as a Humanistic Enterprise." *Sexual and Relationship Therapy* 21 (2006): 359–75.

Toates, F. M. *How Sexual Desire Works*. Cambridge, UK: Cambridge University Press, 2014.

Tolman, Deborah L. *Dilemmas of Desire: Teenage Girls Talk About Sexuality*. Cambridge, MA: Harvard University Press, 2002.

Valenti, Jessica. *Sex Object: A Memoir*. New York: Dey Street, 2016.

Veaux, Franklin, and Eve Rickert. *More than Two: A Practical Guide to Ethical Polyamory*. Portland, OR: Thorntree Press, 2014.

Waller, Robert J. *The Bridges of Madison County*. New York: Grand Central, 1992.

Watter, Daniel. Clinical Case Presentation: "The Relationship Between Death-Anxiety and Sexual Behavior: An Alternative View of Sexual Addiction." SSTAR 38th Annual Meeting, Baltimore, April 6, 2013.

Weber, Jill P. *Having Sex, Wanting Intimacy: Why Women Settle for One-Sided Relationships*. Lanham, MD: Rowman and Littlefield, 2013.

Weiner, Linda, and Constance Avery-Clark. "Sensate Focus: Clarifying the Masters and Johnson's Model." *Sexual and Relationship Therapy* 29, no. 3 (2014): 307–19.

———. *Sensate Focus in Sex Therapy: The Illustrated Manual*. New York: Routledge, 2017.

Winnicott, Donald W. *The Maturational Processes and the Facilitating Environment: Studies in the Theory of Emotional Development*, edited by Masud M. Khan. London: Hogarth Press and the Institute of Psycho-Analysis, 1965.

Yates, Alayne. *Sex Without Shame: Encouraging the Child's Healthy Sexual Development*. New York: William Morrow, 1978.

Zilbergeld, Bernie. *The New Male Sexuality*, rev. ed. New York: Bantam, 1999. Originally published in 1978 as *Male Sexuality*.

Zoldbrod, Aline P. *SexSmart: How Your Childhood Shaped Your Sexual Life and What to Do about It*. Otsego, MI: PageFree, 2005.

Zylowska, Lidia. *The Mindfulness Prescription for Adult ADHD*. Boston: Trumpeter, 2012.

Acknowledgments

Todd Shuster, my agent at Aevitas Creative, believed in this project from the beginning and guided it to completion with wisdom and grace. I've been extremely lucky to have him in my corner.

Elias Altman, Erica Bauman, Jennifer Gates, and Sarah Levitt at Aevitas Creative offered valuable input. Jane von Mehren made extensive suggestions on the proposal and helped put it into its final form.

Jennifer Weis, my editor at St. Martin's Press, improved the manuscript far beyond what I could have envisioned at the start. To her I owe enduring thanks.

Publishers Sally Richardson, Jennifer Enderlin, and Laura Clark at St. Martin's Press took a chance on an unpublished doctor, and tolerated his repeated bouts of stubbornness. Sylvan Creekmore pulled it all together on deadline and made it seem easy. Young Jin Lim provided the beautiful cover design.

Lisa Tener and Sandra Beckwith gave me expert coaching and

assistance throughout. Julie Silver's Harvard Writer's Workshop provided much-needed insights into the publishing world.

Colleagues Margie Nichols and Jack Pula gave valuable guidance at an early stage of this book's development. Lori Brotto, Peggy Kleinplatz, Marta Meana, and Linda Weiner generously agreed to discuss their work with me, and later helped make sure all relevant parts of the text and notes were accurate.

Harold Bronheim, Sallie Foley, and Nathan Kravis made detailed comments on the manuscript. Michael Bader, Ruth Cohn, Betty Dodson, Carol Ellison, Jack Drescher, Kathryn Hall, Ian Kerner, Marty Klein, Joe Kort, Harriet Lerner, Pat Love, Barry McCarthy, Tammy Nelson, Gina Ogden, Esther Perel, Chris Ryan, David Scharff, Julia Serano, Leonore Tiefer, Deborah Tolman, and Daniel Watter gave helpful feedback.

Deborah Berry, Megan Fleming, Sylvia Rosenfeld, William Picker, and the late Carolynn Hillman provided essential support early on. Marianne Brandon, Pamela Madsen, Wednesday Martin, and Tammy Nelson gave generously of their time and knowledge.

Hillary Snyder, Michael Snyder, Natalie and Gilbert Snyder, Shulamis and Norbi Moskovits, Brocha Teichman, and Tzipora and Steven Kalish all provided unflagging support.

My wife Bluma Snyder showered me with more love and acceptance than I could possibly deserve, and graciously accepted the deprivations of marriage to a doctor and author.

Our children Julian and Lily waited patiently for their father to finish his book, helped cheer him up at crucial moments, and have been an unending source of *nachas* and delight.

It is my heartfelt prayer that someday, if they wish, they will find partners as wonderful as their mother.